The Answer is in Your Bloodtype

PERSONAL NUTRITION USA, INC.
PUBLISHER
P.O. BOX 951479
LAKE MARY, FL 32795-1479

Personal Nutrition USA, Inc.

THE ANSWER IS IN YOUR
BLOODTYPE

For more information on this subject, please visit our website at:

www.4blood.com

This book is not intended as a substitute for the medical recommendations of physicians or other healthcare providers. It is intended to offer information to help the reader cooperate with physicians and health professionals in a mutual quest for optimum good health. The identities of the people described in the appendix or otherwise have been changed to protect their confidentiality.

Information provided in reference to medical diagnosis, treatment, and research reflect the view of the authors and should not be taken as medical opinion. In cases of medical issues, an individual should always check with his or her personal physician.

The publisher and the authors are not responsible for any goods and/or services offered or referred to in this book, and expressly disclaim all liability in connection with the fulfillment of orders for any such goods or services, and for any damage, loss, or expense to person or property arising out of or relating to them.

The diet plans presented here are not intended for anyone with kidney problems or for pregnant women or women trying to get pregnant. Readers who are on medication to control cholesterol, blood pressure, fluid retention, or blood sugar or who have an abnormal heart rhythm or have had a heart attack within the last one year must not under any circumstances begin their diet without a physician's guidance and close supervision. Even other readers, however, should consult a physician regarding their individual needs before starting any diet or fitness program.

TABLE OF CONTENTS

ISBN 0-9670125-0-3

Published by: Personal Nutrition USA, Inc.
                 P.O. Box 951479
                 Lake Mary, FL 32795-1479
                 Toll Free (888)41-BLOOD, Fax (407)260-5112

Library of Congress Cataloging-in-Publication Data

Joseph Christiano, A.P.P.T.

Steven M. Weissberg, M.D.

"The Answer is in Your Bloodtype"

ACKNOWLEDGMENTS

To J.J. Messenger, who conceived the Theories of Longevity and Compatibility, and provided the necessary means to do the ongoing research. Without his dedication and perseverance this project would not have been possible.

To Joseph Christiano, author, motivational speaker, educator, internationally recognized fitness expert, believer, and proponent of the diet, exercise, supplementation, and theories upon which this book has been written.

The authors and publisher of this book wish to acknowledge the seminal work of Dr. Peter J. D'Adamo in the field of blood type and nutrition, and his book Eat Right For Your Type (with Catherine Whitney, G.P. Putnam's Sons 1996). This book is not approved, licensed, or endorsed by Dr. D'Adamo.

To the patients, volunteers, medical providers, research assistants, and participants who contributed so much of their time and efforts to this noble cause - Thank You.

Steven M. Weissberg, M.D.

How often have you heard of a newborn that spits up, cries, or won't take a bottle? The anxious parents take the baby to the pediatrician and what does s/he do? S/he changes the formula from regular milk to soymilk and the baby does fine. This baby has not yet had a chance to eat hot dogs, hamburgers, pizza, and other items in a typical diet, yet the baby cannot tolerate the milk. Why?

The infant's digestive system knows instinctively what is good and what is not. Adults have these same instincts, but over time they are discarded or ignored. We can learn much from the infant. He cannot protect himself, but his body is designed to protect him automatically.

We, on the other hand, eat foods that are not good for us over and over again because they taste good and we like them. When the side effects set in we take an antacid, or some other elixir, and hope to get over the episode as quickly as possible. What we should be doing is listening to our bodies, as they are telling us these foods are not good for us.

Our minds say we want to eat this or that food, but internally our bodies are struggling to metabolize them, leading to indigestion, bloating, and gaseous distention. But this is not the whole story. These improper foods are polluting and thickening our blood, depressing our immune systems, and raising our risks for heart disease, cancer, diabetes, weight gain, high blood pressure, stroke, and heart attack.

But it doesn't have to be this way. The human body is a sophisticated and intricate organism that requires the proper fuel and exercise to be its best. And what is best for you may not be best for your spouse, children, parents, or friends. This is because humans are not generic. There are four blood types in humans, and each blood type requires its own diet and exercise to be its best.

After you have read this book you will understand the differences and significance of how your blood type influences your everyday life. You will find that within most families individuals have different blood types, and why. You will understand why some members of your family are at higher risk than others, and why so many individuals die young, while others live to a ripe old age. You will understand why you may be drawn to a mate or friend, and how best to find your perfect mate.

You will learn what foods are best for you and how to live your maximum life span. You will learn how to achieve your optimal weight and forget dieting forever. You will know what the researchers of this book discovered, namely:

<u>THERE IS A DIRECT LINK BETWEEN BLOODTYPE, DIET, DISEASE, COMPATIBILITY, AND LONGEVITY.</u>

Many books have been written about diet and disease, but there has never been a book addressing blood type in relation to compatibility and longevity. J. J. Messenger conceived these two theories as a theoretical hypothesis. The research on longevity and compatibility has never been published before ... not anywhere, by anyone. We believe these theories will become more significant as useful tools for the 21st century.

Data were collected from over 5000 individuals, and were sorted, collated, and placed on charts and graphs so they could be analyzed more easily. This book is the outgrowth of that research. The research uncovered what the conventional medical community and all others had overlooked, namely, the link between blood type, diet, disease, compatibility, and longevity.

After you have read this book, analyzed the data, followed your common sense, and related the information enclosed to yourself and your family, we believe your life will be changed forever. That is no small claim, but we guarantee it!

So we urge you to keep an open mind as you read this fascinating book. And while you're at it, may we suggest that for several weeks you make a few adjustments in accordance with the suggested food lists and exercise regimen, and see if you don't feel better, have more energy, and experience a general feeling of well being. Remember that you have nothing to lose and everything to gain. **It's your life; make the most of it. Good luck and good health!**

Steven M. Weissberg, M.D.

Steven M. Weissberg, M.D., F.A. C.O.G., Board Certified Obstetrician-Gynecologist, with a special interest in Sports Medicine, is a practitioner for over thirty years, and physician of choice to many international celebrities. Based in Miami, Florida, Dr. Weissberg has distinguished himself in the areas of health, sports nutrition, and fertility.

Overseer of the clinical research team who accomplished the groundbreaking research of "The Answer is in Your Bloodtype", Dr. Weissberg is the Medical Director of Team FootWorks Walkers, and author of the column "Ask Dr. Steve", which appears regularly in a nationally published sports newsletter. His other professional writings have been published in over 20 medical journals, professional publications and lay literature, and the research in this book has earned him the nomination for the prestigious Seale-Harris award for his substantial contribution and research in the fields of health and nutrition.

Joseph Christiano, author of "My Body...God's Temple", motivational speaker, educator, and internationally recognized fitness trainer, with 35 years in the fields of health and fitness, provided invaluable experience, dedication and research to this noble cause.

Holder of numerous titles, including 1981- Mr. Florida Bodybuilding Champion, 1982- 1st runner-up as Mr. USA and 4th place in the prestigious Mr. America competition. Joe trained the first Miss Florida to win the swimsuit competition in the Miss America Pageant, and winners in the Miss USA, Miss America, and Mrs. America pageants. He also took part in preparing and training the then-to-be Miss Florida and eventually the 1993 Miss America, Leanza Cornett.

J.J. Messenger is the individual responsible for the Theories of Longevity and Compatibility. These two theories have never been written about by anyone, anywhere, except in this book. J.J. is a working model and proponent of the diet, exercise, supplementation, and theories of this book.

In the early part of this century, the brightest of all men came forth with a theory that was misunderstood, discredited and thought to be outright crazy. It took many years before the second individual on earth even understood what he was thinking, no less proving that what he said was true.

In 1919, in response to a student's question about how he would have reacted if his theory of general relativity had not been confirmed experimentally, he answered:

"THE THEORY IS CORRECT ANYWAY"

Albert Einstein

So, for all those who are ready to discredit, disbelieve and attempt to undermine the findings of this book, especially the Theory of Longevity and the Theory of Compatibility, we feel sorry for them.

THE THEORIES OF LONGEVITY AND COMPATIBILITY
ARE CORRECT

Considering the single most important issue concerning our physical life, one must agree that it is the condition of our health, which stands alone. Many people are oblivious to the potential health related consequences both present and future by simply ignoring the warnings or symptoms of the seemingly obvious declining condition of their health. Modern day man has fallen prey to the demands of his fast-paced, stress-filled life style causing him to place more effort, and in many cases, more value in other areas of his life as priorities, while foregoing his health. In certain instances it can't be helped or at least until our wavering health demands our attention. Whereas in most situations, it is simply a matter of negligence that forces our modern man to live with a slightly less than desirable quality of life.

I realize one cannot argue with the family man who finds it necessary to 'pound the pavement' hour after long hour to support his family. Or the sacrificial mother/wife, who forgoes her own self interests (health included), even to the point of feeling guilty for the very thought of doing something for herself, for the welfare of her family.

But with great emphasis placed on the viability and necessity of healthy bodily functions and performance, whether cognizant of the present condition of our health and its potential future, or simply being unaware, the condition of our health is absolutely the key to a greater or lesser quality of life. Therefore, a measure of effort is a must for improving and maintaining good health. It will be 'impaired' health that brings down the curtain in our life causing everything to come to a screeching halt.

NO MORE SUGAR BLUES OR HYPOGLYCEMIA

For the greater part of my life I had always been a healthy person but for several years I had realized that something was going haywire with my health. It wasn't until 1986 that I began experiencing severe bouts of low levels of energy, lacking mental focus, even nervousness and irritability on a regular basis. Submerged in my new private one-on-one fitness business, with all the hours, commitment and stress that it demanded, I started experiencing what I call 'crashing'.

I found myself 'crashing' on a daily basis. In fact, I could set my watch to the times throughout each day that I would crash. Like clockwork it occurred every morning at 10:00 am and in the afternoons at 3:00 pm. It became my greatest nightmare. It interfered with everything in my life. Crashing, as I call it, refers to when a person experiences extreme light headedness, tiredness, sleepiness, sometimes anxiety, irritability, mental depression (when there was no apparent reason). Generally this is followed by the uncontrollable cravings for sweets. Keep in mind, there is a difference between a candy bar grabbing your hand and saying, "eat me", then when you intentionally reach for it because you're in the mood for something sweet. These symptoms that I was experiencing were in fact the warning signs telling me that something was wrong with my health.

I recall many times going to my favorite Chinese restaurant for lunch. After returning to the studio and resuming my workout sessions with my clients, it was within an hour to two that I was almost falling asleep on my feet. I started feeling tired, yawning as if I hadn't slept in weeks while finding it difficult keeping mentally focused. I could not figure out what was wrong. BUT SOMETHING WAS!

On another occasion I had been out with my wife Lori for a drive. We happened to be enjoying a couple of candy bars (big splurge) while talking and driving around. Later that evening I pulled into a service station to fill up. I asked Lori if she would pump the gas, as I was extremely tired, and EXTREMELY DRAINED OF ENERGY. By the time she got back into the car, I was passed out at the wheel. SOMETHING WAS WRONG!!

After having experienced these severe bouts with low blood sugar and thousands more like them, I decided to see a doctor for a glucose test. The test revealed that after ingesting a highly concentrated form of sugar, my blood sugar had shot up as expected, but instead of returning back and leveling out, it continued to tumble down causing me to crash. I was hypoglycemic. I had been experiencing these severe bouts of low blood sugar to the point that my tolerance for glucose (simple sugar) was zilch.

I had read a few books referred by physicians as well as following their eating plans for controlling my hypoglycemic condition. Much that I read and applied fell far from ridding this condition. There was too much controversy with each of their positions taken. Meanwhile, I was still battling with this dilemma. Well, this condition went on for the next ten years. During those years I had arranged then rearranged and then readjusted my selections of foods in hopes of discovering a combination that would put this monster to bed.

The most success I experienced was when I applied the glycemic index concept for food selections. For example, I had removed all white flour products in exchange for wheat but still no satisfactory results. I added some milk to my diet for a protein source but to no avail, I was still experiencing low blood sugar or "crashing". I was baffled, bewildered and hated this nightmare that I had been experiencing for so many years.

It wasn't until June of 1997 that I discovered the theory of eating foods that were compatible to my blood type that had revolutionized my entire approach to eating. Eating foods that are compatible to one's blood type is what I have come to believe and embrace ever since. In my experience this is unequivocally the most sound, scientifically based, and comprehensive way of eating.

As I learned about which foods were compatible to my blood type and which ones were not I began applying this new found knowledge. I began experiencing some very wonderful things. I learned that wheat flour products that had been suggested as 'good' foods for controlling hypoglycemia were an 'avoid' and a poison to my body. I also learned that the grains, bread, and milk that were recommended as 'good' for controlling hypoglycemia were 'avoid' for my blood type. These very foods that were recommended as 'good' were actually the foods that contributed to my blood sugar problems.

It was not long before I experienced something that I had not experienced in almost 15 years, NO MORE CRASHING. I had found how to win the battle of suffering from low blood sugar. I had gained a whole new grip on life and my once impaired health problem went out the window. I had won the battle in only a couple of days by simply eating foods that were compatible to my blood type.

As I changed my approach to eating only foods that were highly beneficial and neutral for my blood type, not only did I overcome my battle with hypoglycemia (of which I have not experienced any more 'crashing'), but also I lost a significant percent of body fat. While increasing my lean weight (muscle) I acquired a better quality of body composition, also.

To my understanding and experience, I was constantly amazed by the relationship that foods have with the different blood types. Because of being a blood type O, I had learned that my digestive system was compatible for digesting red meat due to a naturally high level of stomach acid. This in fact made eating red meat a primary source of protein and considered highly beneficial. I had discovered that I am a meat eater.

There is a particular restaurant that my wife and I enjoy dining at. This restaurant provided a bucket of peanuts that one could indulge themselves with before their meal. I noticed that every time after eating those peanuts I would experience a slight upset stomach.

In retrospect, I found it totally fascinating that as I began to understand the connection that foods have with the different blood types that me, being blood type O would find peanuts to be an 'avoid' food, ultimately causing my upset stomach.

So now the old adage; "YOU ARE WHAT YOU EAT" can be improved upon once you learn to "EAT WHAT YOU ARE".™

Well, until this point I normally ate red meat only once every month or so simply because I was concerned about my blood lipids, etc. But now I found myself consuming a pound or more per day. I felt stronger, my energy levels were constant, I felt great, and my crashing days were over. And all this time I thought I was in a good healthy condition.

After approximately 6 months of eating red meat as my primary source of protein on a daily basis, I decided to see what was going on, on the inside. So I scheduled some blood work to determine the condition of my blood lipids, etc. When I received my test results I was astounded with the results. All my statistics were in the low normal ranges or better (and that's with wolfing down a couple of pounds of red meat a day for 6 months straight).

THE COMPLETE PACKAGE

Because I had become a true believer and embraced this approach to healthier and wiser eating, I also have become proactive or have been eating (practicing) this way for approximately a year and a half. By simply changing my food selections I have become a recipient of the many benefits that are available to all that follow this approach to eating. I've experienced new levels of energy, constant blood sugar levels, very low cholesterol levels, feel great and even enjoy some of the cosmetic benefits like more muscularity and leanness that happens as a by-product when your health is improved.

Being the advocate of physical exercise and its rewards that I am, I am also aware of the greater demands that are placed on the body because of it. For this reason there is a greater requirement for additional nutrition.

In our attempts for being healthier individuals, most of us realize the importance of nutrition. Probably most do not know the value and importance of minerals and vitamins for maintaining good health. For example, in a perfect world, we would obtain our mineral and vitamin source from the foods we eat such as: veggies, fruits, and grains. But in our not so perfect world we as a nation face a serious problem when it comes to the nutrient values found in our foods. Because of the way the soil, water and air have been polluted with chemicals, pesticides, fertilizers, waste materials, etc., our good old natural sources for helping us stay healthier are no longer able to provide us with the total nutrient values they once could.

The following information was published in Senate document 264 back in 1936:

SENATE DOCUMENT 264

"The alarming fact is that the foods (fruits, vegetables and grains) now being raised on millions of acres of land that no longer contain enough of certain minerals are starving us– no matter how much of them we eat. No man today can eat enough fruits and vegetables to supply his system with the minerals he requires for perfect health, because his stomach isn't big enough to hold them. The truth is that our foods vary enormously in value, and some of them aren't worth eating as food. Our physical well being is more directly dependent upon the minerals we take into our systems than upon calories or vitamins or upon the precise proportions of starch, protein or carbohydrates we consume."

With sobering findings like these, one realizes that with our very best effort in selecting foods in their most natural state, we are running around nutritionally deficient.

For this very reason and other factors such as stressful lifestyles, physical exercise, proper bodily function, human performance, etc., taking dietary supplementation regularly plays an important role for staying healthy.

A synergistic component that helps in meeting the nutritional requirements necessary for good health and that works alongside with eating is taking dietary supplements. But as we make advancements such as in the understanding of how foods relate to our blood type, likewise, advancements have been made toward useful dietary supplements.

Having spent the last 35 years both personally and professionally in the health and fitness industry, my awareness of these issues had always led me to learning and discovering new and improved-upon methods and procedures that would play a vital role in staying healthy.

As I have already attested to embracing this approach to eating foods that are compatible to blood types, I was in search of one or two more components that would make this dietary approach toward healthier living complete.

As critical as it is for our health to eat foods that are compatible to our blood type, it only makes sense then, that we take dietary supplements that are also compatible with our blood type. As a matter of fact, how about a protein powder mix drink that also is compatible to all blood types?

And so with this desire and passion for learning for my better understanding and providing good information, systems and products that would benefit others, I found a company called Personal Nutrition USA, Inc., that has done just that. This company has formulated a multi-vitamin and mineral supplement as well as a protein powder drink that are both blood type specific. They also make a protein drink that all blood types can drink.

The beauty of all this is that now there is a complete package, a complete scientific approach to staying healthy through eating foods and taking dietary supplements that are compatible to blood type.

Besides selecting foods which are most compatible for my blood type, I make sure I'm meeting all my nutritional requirements by daily supplementing with Personal Vitamins™, a multi-vitamin, mineral and herbal supplement. In addition, I include Personal Protein™, a high quality protein shake as an anabolic snack or compliment to a meal.

This approach to healthier living makes for a very individualized and personal dietary package for everybody.

SPREADING THE GOOD NEWS

I found my personal experiences from eating foods that are compatible to my blood type very beneficial and worthy of explanation. As a professional fitness trainer, educator and speaker, I encounter people from all walks of life, backgrounds, professions and health conditions. Many people I meet suffer from obesity, high blood pressure, irritable bowel syndrome, poor digestion, constipation, hypoglycemia, high cholesterol and more. As a conduit of information, I thought it criminal not to share the 'good news' and concept of eating foods and taking dietary supplements what were compatible to their blood types.

As I shared my excitement and as much information as I could with my clients I could sense their individual attention and interest. I knew that if I could get their attention and help guide them with this approach to eating, they would experience a whole new level of well being, energy, fat loss and more.

In Orlando, Florida, my wife Lori and I conduct Fitness and Fellowship group fitness classes as one component of our fitness vocation. It's a program where we provide an exercise program that is progressive in nature and lasts for 6 weeks. During those 6 weeks our students are educated on the importance of combining regular exercise, sensible eating (according to blood type) and dietary supplementation.

It has been our experience without fail that those who adhere to eating foods that are compatible with their blood type, and avoid eating the 'avoid' foods, which are not compatible, experience wonderful results. The following are just some of the statistics and testimonials of actual students that attend our program.

STUDENT #1

Marsha - A 41 year old wife and mother

"I have really enjoyed the fitness and fellowship 6-week program. I have learned how to eat healthy by eating according to my blood type. It's a way of life for me now and not hard to stick to because I can eat plenty of food and lose weight naturally. I don't feel full or sluggish after eating because I eat small snacks all through the day. It has also been a great help learning to keep the protein level up above the carbohydrates. I have more energy and I don't feel like I am carrying around the water weight. My complexion is much cleaner; my blood pressure has stayed in the normal range. I have lost inches and I feel much better about myself. I am on the right healthy track. Thanks."

Now lets look at the results:

	9/14/98	10/12/98		9/14/98	10/12/98
Shoulders	37	39	Thighs/R	22	21 1/4
Chest	34	34 1/4	Thighs/L	22	21 1/2
Arms/R	12 1/2	11	Height	5'1"	
Arms/L	12	11	Weight	131	129
Waist	32 1/2	30 1/2	Body Fat %	31 3/4	26 1/4
Hips	39	37 1/2			

Total loss

Overall Inches 7 3/4, Weight lost 2 lbs., Body fat lost 5%

The results that Marsha experienced happened within only 4 weeks. These results are excellent for such a very short period of time. The combination of eating according to her blood type A and taking dietary supplementation, including Personal Protein and Personal Vitamins and proper exercise has provided these results. (see Chapter VIII on exercise).

STUDENT #2

Laurie - 49 year old wife, mother, and professional

"Knowing I am a type O gives me freedom to enjoy more red meats a little more often than normally I would have in the past. Eating according to my blood type has made my former eating habits do a complete flip-flop."

	9/17/98	10/15/98
Shoulders	36 1/2	36 1/2
Bust	34 1/2	34 1/2
Arms/ L	10 1/2	10 3/4
Arms/ R	10 1/2	10 3/4
Waist	27 1/2	26 1/2
Hips	38"	35 1/2
Thighs/ R	21 3/4	21 1/2
Thighs/ L	21 3/4	21 1/2
Calves	13 3/4	13 1/4
Weight	124	120
Body Fat %	28%	22%

Total Loss

Overall 5 1/2 inches, 4 lbs. Weight loss, 6% body fat loss

These results were accomplished in only 4 weeks. Her success was the combination of eating foods that were compatible to her blood type, taking dietary supplements, and proper exercise.

STUDENT #3

Jeanette W. - 29 year old wife, mother and professional

"Believe it or not, I felt like I had mud flowing through my veins. I honestly could go to bed at 5:30 (1/2 hr. after work) and sleep until 7am the next morning. It must be the eating according to blood type B foods and Personal Vitamins™ because since I started, I still have energy. The cravings for sweets are almost gone."

	9/17/98	10/15/98
Shoulders	47	45 1/2
Bust	43 1/2	42 3/4
Arms/ R	14 1/2	13 1/4
Arms/ L	13 1/2	13 1/4
Waist	33 3/4	32 1/2
Hips	42	40 1/2
Thighs/ R	25 1/2	24 3/4
Thighs/ L	25	24 3/4
Weight	170	165
Body Fat%	37 1/2	34%

Total loss

Overall 8 1/2", Weight loss 5 lbs., Body Fat loss 3%

Jeanette made this great progress in just 4 weeks. The combination of eating according to her blood type, taking dietary supplements, and proper exercise allowed her to achieve these results.

TESTIMONIALS

David B., 63 year old construction worker, Blood Type O

"My energy level is better than ever. I love eating Ezekiel bread. I knew I always loved steak but I did not know why, until I understood about my blood type. I feel like a kid again."

Carolyn - 52 year old mom, Blood Type O

"Thanks for giving my mind back to me. I started eating according to my blood type, taking Personal Protein drinks and Personal Vitamins and in two days I have not felt like taking a nap in the middle of the day. My children are amazed at my new energy."

CeCe - 41 year old wife, mom, Blood Type A

"I am convinced that eating according to my blood type along with adding Personal Protein drinks and Personal Vitamins that my body has taken on a whole new improved condition. My struggle with low blood sugar has disappeared as well as the cravings for sweets. My energy has not been like this ever. It has changed my entire family's health also."

THE BALANCING ACT

You have read just a few testimonials of real people who have shared their exciting results and newfound grip on life. Some shared their positive experiences when changing their eating habits to eating foods that were compatible with their blood type. Then some mentioned how protein and vitamins played an important component in their journey for becoming healthier.

A single link of chain is in and of itself neither strong nor weak, but certainly limited until it is connected with additional links. Once connected, you have created a synergy that is capable of pulling or towing heavy loads such as trucks or automobiles that the single link of chain could not accomplish.

So similar is the success of becoming healthier and staying healthier. Just as our success stories are shared, much success can be accomplished through dietary changes alone. Improvements are experienced when dietary supplementation is added to a diet. Just a single protein drink per day can make a big difference in our energy, but like the single link of chain, there needs to be the synergy of all the components (links) to obtain optimum health and bodily function.

Without reiterating on what has already been mentioned in this book regarding the importance of regular exercise, it is scientifically as well as medically proven that regular exercise promotes and assists greater health. A warning from the Surgeon General's 1996 report on the benefits of physical activity should be a wake up call to all, **"Physical inactivity may be detrimental to your health."**

In search for a better quality of health and life it's the synergy of the three major components compatible to your blood chemistry working in concert with each other that will produce optimum health: regular exercise, sensible eating, and dietary supplementation.

To help you with your dietary journey refer to:
TIPS FOR KEEPING THINGS SIMPLE, on page 247

If you look at your family tree and find that close family members have died at an early age of either heart disease or cancer, there is a very high likelihood that your blood type is A or AB. This is because most cancers are associated with group A, as are clotting diseases, including blood clots, which in many cases lead to coronary heart disease and fatal heart attacks. As the person who pushed this research from the beginning, I would ask you the reader, to examine my case history.

My father's entire family was Blood Type A, and they died young. My father died at age 59, his mother at 32, his father at 64, his sister at 66, and my uncle, who was very athletic and lived the longest, at age 71. My brother, also Type A, had a heart attack at 47 and died of heart failure at age 50. All were struck down with heart attacks, some with warning, some without.

My mother's entire family is Blood Type B, and they have lived considerably longer. Not one has ever died of a heart attack. Despite chronic illnesses on my mother's side, she is alive and well today at 74, as are her sisters, at 79 and 85.

I was 47 when my brother died, and from what I could see I didn't have long to live. My blood pressure was elevated and I had been prescribed medication, but was reluctant to take it. I was determined to find out what was happening in my family and why. While pursuing an investigation, I started an exercise program, stopped eating meat, and began to eat only fruits, vegetables, grains and fish.

I started having my blood checked regularly, and although there was improvement, the results were not dramatic. I donated blood at the Red Cross, because I'd read that this could reduce heart attack risk by 85%. In the process, they provided my blood type free and advised me that it was very rare. In fact my blood type was the most rare-Type AB-representing only two to four percent of all the people in the world. I was confused and amazed all at the same time.

Was it coincidence that everyone in my family of blood type A had died of heart disease at an early age? Was it coincidence that everyone in my family of blood type B was still alive? And how was it I was a different blood type from my father and mother and brother. I was driven to find out what was happening and why.

I started talking to all the people I'd meet about their blood type, disease profiles, and whether their parents were alive or not. I wanted to know why half my family died young, and not the other half. Every time I met another AB I would ask if one of the parents had died young. The overwhelming number of ABs had lost one parent, the Type A, usually from heart disease or cancer.

A strong pattern started to emerge and I knew I was on to something. Why was the A type dying before the B type? And in cases where an A was married to an O, why again was the A type dying so much younger, while the Os appeared to be living much longer. The more I looked at the data, the more I knew it wasn't a coincidence.

Finally I met Steven M. Weissberg, MD, and explained my theories of longevity and compatibility. He embraced the idea of further research based upon the data already collected. This book is the culmination of that research. My goal was and still is to help people and extend life. I hope this book saves, or extends your life or that of a loved one you know.

J. J. MESSENGER

At the dawn of man it is presumed that the orginal blood type was O and that meat was the primary source of protein. But because of migration to different regions and environments, man had to adjust accordingly. Just as animals have adapted to survive, so has man. Through adaptation the development of the other three blood types emerged. The hunters adapted to vegetarian, or A Type. When new food sources became available, again man adapted, resulting in the B and AB blood types.

It has also been found that given the right diet, each blood type can extend life expectancy up to twenty years. If that surprises you, read on.

It has been shown that blood types have a great deal to do with physical characteristics, personality traits, sexual preferences, vocational likes and dislikes, and even compatibility inclinations. Have you ever wondered why people with seemingly equal life style and diet to others appear to be healthier, have more energy, age more gracefully, and have an overall fuller life?

Maybe it is not metabolism, will power, or genetics per se, but something else at work. That something else led to many questions, perhaps some of which you have been wondering about.

- Did you know that research has conclusively shown a direct link between blood type, diet, disease, and longevity?

- Did you know that research has shown a direct link between blood type and your most compatible mate or spouse?

- Did you know that high carbohydrate diets increase water retention (three grams water/H2O to every gram of glycogen-stored muscle sugar), making you look soft and puffy, as well as reducing your body's ability to burn fat?

- Did you know that 70% of your body's energy, when at rest (not exercising), comes from fat, not carbohydrate? (But high carbohydrate diets stop you from accessing the fat).

- Did you know that high insulin levels in your body, from eating lots of carbohydrates, lower your body's anabolic response, growth hormone secretion, immune response, and boost fat storing enzymes, all at the same time?

- Did you know that obesity in America has risen 33% over the last ten years despite a decrease in overall fat consumption?

- Did you know that nearly 60% of overweight Americans who manage to lose weight regain it all within a year?

- Did you know that 75% of the American population is unable to benefit from a high carbohydrate diet?

- Did you know that certain fats are good for you, and increase fat burning and metabolic rate?

If any or all of this information is news to you, then this book will answer the above questions in detail, and explain why each blood type requires different food sources, exercise regimens, and the proper balance of each to stay fit and healthy. The goal is to live to your potential life span.

It's your life; live it to the fullest.

CHAPTER II

AN EXPLANATION OF
BLOOD GROUPS IN HUMANS

There are four blood types in humans: A, B, AB and O. Type O represents approximately 50% of the population of the world; Type A, 40%; Type B, approximately 8% and Type AB, only 2%. Each blood type group evolved as a result of environmental conditions and available food supplies. The oldest and original blood group was Type O. Considering that animal protein was most plentiful it is consistent that individuals of Blood Type O would do well on a diet high in protein, supplemented by fruits and vegetables.

As we explain later, our research shows that individuals of Blood Type O have the longest life span. This is attributable, in part, to their ability to eat meat protein and their strong immune systems and stomach acid, which can metabolize almost any food.

The first mutation from Type O was Type A. When primarily meat eaters moved, migrated, or were forced to leave the territories where meat was most abundant – to areas of the globe where meat was scarce (or less plentiful) – an adjustment was made to adapt to new and different food sources. Thus, Type A individuals over time adjusted to a diet rich in fruits and vegetables, with little or no meat. It is for this reason that almost all Type A individuals thrive on a vegetarian diet. Those Type As who eat the typical American diet typically die younger because their bodies do not properly metabolize meat or dairy products, which are loaded with saturated fat. Coupled with a predisposition toward thick blood, type As are particularly susceptible to heart disease, high blood pressure, anemia and a host of other ailments.

One exception lies within Type A. There are A1 and A2 Types. As A2 was the first adaptation of Type O, it carries many of the genetic characteristics of Type O, especially in the area of muscle mass and the ability to eat a wider variety of foods than Type A1. In our research, we found individuals who were A2 by virtue of their muscle mass, but had to eat vegetarian to stay healthy. Those who did not follow a vegetarian diet invariably developed high blood pressure or heart disease. We also found other A2 types who did not exhibit muscle mass but were able to tolerate meat proteins with little or no evident side effects.

Type B was the third blood type to emerge. Type B individuals can eat both meat and dairy, and is the only blood type that does this well. Also, Type B individuals live the second longest, in part because of their variety of diet choices, which is more liberal than Types A or AB.

Type AB is the newest blood group and it is estimated that it came into existence approximately 2,000 years ago. There is little data about AB, but it is believed that it came about as a result of mixing of individuals of Types A and B. On the surface this seems logical, genetically speaking. Since Types A and B are both dominant traits one would expect that if a Type A mixes with a Type B, the outcome should be A or B, which occurs in the vast majority of cases. But for reasons yet unknown, in a very small number of cases, approximately one in nine times, the new distinct AB blood type emerged. Type AB may represent the ultimate adaptation by virtue of the fact that man no longer needs to hunt for food, and because both A and B are more resistant to diseases that once decimated the O populations of the world throughout history. Since AB is more resistant to typhoid, plague, smallpox, diphtheria, cholera, and malaria, the merging of the two dominant genes could represent the latest adaptation to insure the survival of the human race. Only time will tell.

With this overview of the four blood types, we can now look into the details that set them apart, their different strengths and weaknesses, the reasons for compatibility (or incompatibility), and the individual longevity of each group relative to the others.

BLOOD TYPE O

Individuals of Type O blood have the thinnest blood, strongest immune systems (with the exception of some diseases) strongest stomach acid, and live the longest of all the blood types at present.

The authors of this book base this opinion on the research data collected, but attribute much of this longevity upon the Type Os ability to metabolize almost any food as a result of high stomach acid, and naturally thin blood.

Genetically, stomach acid was needed to break down the high protein diets on which our original ancestors thrived. This very strong acid is required to break down protein completely, and since animal protein was one of our original food sources, man adapted to survive. And as food sources changed the Type O was able to adapt to metabolizing almost any food because of this strong stomach acid.

Also, since the staple diet in the United States has been meat and potatoes, the Type O individual has done quite well on this diet, while other blood types did not. A negative side affect of strong stomach acid is it can lead to ulcers when no food is available, or when food is not eaten at regular intervals. This is one reason why Type Os are more prone to stomach ulcers.

Since the ancestors of Type O were hunters, descendants carrying this gene tend to be larger, stronger individuals. This is the product of the adaptation process and the survival of the species. If you must hunt for your food, and you aren't big or strong, your chances for survival would be diminished by the lack of adaptation. That survival was guaranteed precisely because of man's ability to adapt and mutate so as to accommodate different environments with different food sources.

If you were to check the blood types of most competitive body builders, professional athletes, such as football, baseball, basketball, hockey players, and boxers, you would find that an overwhelming number of them are of blood type O. If you check the blood type of the American Indians and Eskimos, who were, and in some cases still are, hunters almost all of them are blood type O.

Excepting the American Indian, another factor contributing to the longevity of blood Type O individuals, at least in the United States, is that the diseases that once killed Type Os by the millions have been all but eradicated. I am referring to typhoid, cholera, smallpox, plague, malaria, and other diseases that exist only in some Third World countries.

In the Middle Ages, and even up to the early part of this century, these diseases wiped out half the populations of Europe and elsewhere. Although individuals of blood type O have very strong immune systems, they are more susceptible to these particular diseases than the other blood types. This is consistent with the mutation of other blood types to insure the survival of the species.

Since so many in the population are blood type O you would expect medical science to concentrate its research on eliminating these diseases. And sure enough, these diseases have been all but eradicated in most countries, including the United States, to the benefit of Type Os.

In fact, if you look at India, a country that still has these diseases, you will find a smaller population of blood type O individuals than in countries that has eliminated these diseases. If you look at Table 2 you will notice that of all the countries in the world India has the smallest number of Type Os as a direct result of the susceptibility to the diseases listed above.

Once you have eliminated the disease factor, it is a known fact that to be nutritionally healthy a person needs to have the essential amino acids, that group of nitrogen-containing, carbon-based organic compounds that serve as the building blocks from which protein (and muscle) are made. All of the essential amino acids are contained naturally in animal protein; thus a Type O eats animal protein, he acquires these essential amino acids, and remains strong and healthy.

However, when Types A and AB eat animal protein, while they may, and we emphasize may, receive their essential amino acids, in the process they are exposing themselves to heart disease and cancer by eating foods that are not compatible with their blood enzymes. Saturated animal fat tends to clog the arteries of As and ABs by virtue of their thicker blood. It is for this reason Types A and AB should obtain their essential amino acids through a combination of foods, namely vegetable and plant protein. To do this requires some planning; what comes naturally to Types Os by way of diet requires much more planning and vigilance by Types A and AB.

We all want to eat right, but for most of us it is a guessing game. Type Os, by and large, can metabolize more food sources as a result of their strong stomach acid than any other blood type. For this reason they more easily acquire proper nutrition with the least amount of effort. All other blood types must acquire proper nutrition with combinations of foods compatible with their lower stomach acid content and blood enzymes.

If the reasons above were not enough to explain why Type Os live longer, let us explain further. Individuals of this blood type lack several blood clotting factors. That is to say, they have the thinnest blood. For this reason, it is suggested that individuals with Type O blood eat foods rich in vitamin K, such as kale, spinach, liver, and egg yolks, which aid in normal clotting. However, the fact that their blood lacks this clotting factor is a plus when it comes to heart disease.

Unlike Type As, who have thick blood that allows fats to build up on artery walls, the thin blood of Type Os is less likely to clot, making it more difficult for plaque to build up. Coupled with their stomach acid, which metabolizes meat protein well, and an enzyme that helps neutralize cholesterol in the intestines, this greatly reduces the incidence of heart disease in Type Os until later years.

As a result of this great metabolizing stomach acid, thinner blood, lack of clotting factor, and ability to eat foods, which provide all the essential amino acids, Type Os also are at a lower risk for cancer. Since most cancers tend to occur in Type As, Os typically dodge this bullet. Some studies even indicate that when Type O individuals do contract heart problems and cancer their survival rates are much higher than Type As, B, and AB individuals.

In our research, we found numerous subjects in their 70s, 80s, and 90s, both men and women of Type O blood, who had no heart disease. At first glance it would seem amazing. But in light of the above, it is predictable. When you consider heart disease and cancer are the number one and number two killers in the United States, and Type Os are the least likely to develop these diseases because of their inherent genetics, it is no wonder so many typically live to a ripe old age.

This is not to say individuals of Type O blood do not get heart disease or cancer, but the research indicates the onset of heart disease is later than for all other blood types. And because most cancers are Type A gene-oriented, when Os do get cancer, it tends not to spread as quickly and can be contained more easily, thereby increasing the mortality life span considerably.

With the lack of a clotting factor and thinner blood, should a Type O individual develop a clot, it is not as life threatening as a Type A with a clot. The Type A individual, who has thick blood, is more likely to experience a life-threatening clot. This is one reason so many Type A individuals die of sudden heart attacks, while Type O individuals may live through a series of heart attacks, but are more likely to die of a stroke when the thin blood does not clot in the brain.

We interviewed many individuals of Type O blood who experienced heart attacks and found many had suffered little or no heart damage. In fact, when they were examined subsequent to the attack, many showed clear arteries with little or no buildup of plaque. This leads us to believe that the attack was either a result of stress, or a severe restriction of the blood vessels, of or around the heart, which subsided when the stress was relieved, or as the result of a temporary clot which dissolved in their thin blood, prior to causing severe heart damage. Individuals of Type A and AB blood are not typically so lucky.

Our research did find that individuals of blood type O were more susceptible to blood disorders, such as hemophilia and leukemia. While both of these blood disorders can be deadly, medical science has come a long way in extending and treating these potential killers. While stroke is not typically considered a blood disorder, it is significant, or life threatening, when the blood does not clot normally. However, our research showed that although Os did suffer from strokes, these tended to be later in life, and many recovered to go on and live long productive lives.

Another area where Os kept showing up in research was arthritis and/or diseases causing swelling and inflammation of the joints. Regarding typical arthritis it appeared that foods causing this condition were white and/or red potatoes, orange juice, and dairy products in general. We found arthritis and joint inflammation in individuals of this blood type, starting in their 20s and following them into old age, to be rampant. Those who ate the least amount of red and white potatoes, dairy, and orange juice appeared to have the least arthritis and related ailments.

On the same note, our research found two related but different diseases that attacked individuals of Type O blood. We are talking about Ankylosing spondylitis, and rheumatoid arthritis. Although the symptoms are similar, in that the joints become inflamed and swollen, the first disease attacks the joints in the spine and is progressive until there is sometimes complete fusion. This disease also tends to run in families.

On the other hand, rheumatoid arthritis is a chronic, systemic inflammatory disease that primarily attacks peripheral joints and surrounding muscles, tendon, ligaments, and blood vessels. While medical science does not know the reason for this disease, we believe the problem lies in improper diet.

This just goes to show that each blood type suffers in a different way, and the Os tend to suffer in a way that is painful but is delayed life threatening, unlike other blood groups.

One other interesting phenomenon we experienced through our interviews was that among older individuals who were still smoking, particularly men over 75, almost every subject was a Type O. For some reason, individuals of all other blood types who previously smoked had quit for health reasons. Only the Type Os were still smoking into their 80s and 90s. Furthermore, almost none of them, in spite of their smoking, had heart disease.

The above is not always true for all individuals of Type O blood, but our research clearly indicated that this blood group appeared to have the greatest threshold for abuse of all other blood types.

Whether it is their thin blood, that tends to be protective against heart disease until later in life, or the fact that cancer is not as likely to attack this blood group, the statistics of longevity are clearly in favor of the Os.

BLOOD TYPE A

The first mutation from blood Type O was A. As stated earlier, there are the A1 and A2 Types. The A2 Type evolved first, and was the first to move from an environment of plentiful animal food to regions where no animals existed, or were not abundant. Since the A2 Type is a partial mutation of Type O, individuals of this trait carry much of the muscle genetics of Os and can eat a variety of animal proteins that A1s cannot tolerate.

It is believed the A2 type developed by mutating partially to a different diet, specifically vegetarian, through migration to areas where meat was not available, then back to places where it was again available. A second theory, which is not fully understood, holds that a partial mutation took place requiring the A2 to maintain muscle for survival reasons, but the mutation did not fully extend to the digestive tract which had already made the adjustment away from meat protein. A third theory would propose that because the A2 was the first mutation from blood type O, that individuals of this blood carry the O recessive gene thereby allowing them many of the characteristics of the O gene, but not to the extent of the dominant O gene individuals. This is still a mystery to anthropologists. Nevertheless, there is no doubt the A blood type is the only partially mutated gene; this does not exist for the other blood types.

The vast majority of Type A individuals are A1. Since these individuals migrated to Europe, Asia and Australia, regions totally different from the plentiful plains of Africa where animal protein was abundant, their systems evolved to survive on food sources, mainly fruits, vegetables and grains. This was totally different than their ancestor Os, who lived primarily on meat proteins and no grains whatsoever. In fact, their mutation is so complete as to be healthy; Type A1s must avoid almost all animal protein in favor of a vegetarian diet.

The interesting diversity of the A type is a true challenge to understand. In fact some of the most muscular individuals we encountered were all A2 types, who maintained their muscle mass on meat protein and not a vegetarian diet. However, the meat-eating subjects, almost to the last, developed heart disease at an early age. They looked strong physically, but internally, they were time bombs. We did find exceptions, but they were just that.

In the United States, meat and potatoes comprise the staple diet. Type As do not tolerate either meat or potatoes well. This is the major reason why Type A individuals live the shortest life span today. When Type As continue to eat meat and potatoes that are inconsistent with their blood enzymes, agglutination, or thickening of their already thick blood, takes place and disaster follows.

If you look at the recommended food list for Blood Type A, you will see more foods inconsistent with the typical American diet than for any other blood type. Constant eating of these latter foods provides fewer nutrients to the body, lowers immune function, and thickens the blood, which leads to heart disease, cancer and earlier death, statistically.

It is precisely for these reasons that Type As are so susceptible and do die of heart disease and cancer in record numbers. The exception is the Japanese, who eat a staple diet of fish, rice and green tea – the perfect diet for individuals of Type A blood. In fact the Japanese life span is longer, as a country, than any other: 78 for men, 83 for women. Their counterparts in the United States who eat the typical American diet live a considerably shorter life span, as the statistics indicate. Knowing this information, the life span of Type As in this country is rather predictable. Let me explain further.

Individuals of Type A blood have the thickest blood of all types. Since the blood is thick as it moves through the arteries and veins, especially after or during periods of sleep, any saturated fat in the bloodstream has an opportunity to deposit itself more easily. When type As eat animal fat, meat or dairy-foods inconsistent with their blood type – their already thick blood agglutinates, or gets thicker and stickier. You don't have to be a rocket scientist to see that any saturated fat now has the opportunity to deposit itself in unwanted places. The thick blood requires the heart to pump harder, inevitably causing high blood pressure, hypertension, an enlarged heart muscle, and an increase in heart disease.

Another downside to Type A blood is that in the adaptation/mutation to a vegetarian diet, Type As lost the stomach acid necessary to metabolize meat protein. In fact, Type As have very low stomach acid by genetic standards; while the low acid accommodates the metabolism of fruits and vegetables, it does a miserable job metabolizing animal protein. This is where type As are in double jeopardy-by consuming foods that agglutinate already thick blood to make it thicker.

Since Type As already have thick blood, this phenomenon only allows the damage from the build-up of plaque on the artery walls to proceed faster, leading to the blood pressure and heart problems mentioned above. The second major issue for Type A, and just as dangerous, is in eating foods that don't metabolize well, causing agglutination, or thicker stickier blood. This in turn lowers immune function, thereby causing or increasing the chances for cancer to develop.

In a society where 40% of the population is Type A, and only five percent of those are true vegetarian, the consequences are catastrophic. Coupled with the fact that researchers agree that most cancers are Type A-related, and the majority of As eat a meat-and-potato diet and a litany of foods unsuitable for their blood type, it is indeed predictable this blood type would be overwhelmed with high blood pressure, heart disease, diabetes, anemia, and cancer.

Another factor that may play a role in the heart/cancer link is stress. Type A individuals seem to be affected more by stress than the other blood groups. It is reasonable to assume that if individuals consistently eat foods not compatible with their blood type, and their immune system is not functioning properly, stress becomes more of a factor than in an individual whose immune system is strong and functioning well. We attribute the stress factor as a great killer of blood type A, in addition to the above, for the following other reasons:

When the brain perceives stress, either from an internal or external trigger, the fight or flight response kicks in. Initially, this reaction stimulates the release of two stress hormones: adrenaline, which is produced by the adrenal glands near the kidneys, and corticotrophin-releasing hormone (CRH), from nerve cells in the hypothalamus, at the base of the brain. CRH then travels to the pituitary gland, where it causes the release of adrenocorticotrophic hormone (ACTH); this triggers the production of cortisol by the adrenal gland.

In response, blood platelets aggregate, immune cells activate, blood sugar rushes to muscles to give them energy, the heart and breathing rate quickens, and blood pressure rises. Cortisol, a steroid hormone that at first sustains the stress response, later slows it down so the body can return to normal functioning.

The obvious problem occurs when an individual of type A blood has this response. His already thick blood, that is even thicker from agglutination, from improper foods, becomes even thicker and subject to dangerous clot forming, by virtue of the flight or fight response. The type A individual is in greater jeopardy of a sudden heart attack from clot forming as a result of the chain reaction of events, normal hormonal responses, or a clot or plaque buildup that may be dislodged as a result of the dramatic and sudden increase of blood pressure. For all of the above reasons we believe more As die more often from sudden heart attacks than any other blood group.

Further, if the individual is subjected to chronic stress, the stress hormones may fail to turn off, and cortisol and other hormones can get out of balance. Instead of providing protection, they may suppress the immune system by interfering with the regular repair and maintenance functions of the body, leaving the individual open to infections and disease, especially cancer.

Therefore, we conclude that individuals of this blood type are at the highest risk for heart disease and cancer, as our mortality tables clearly show, because of their genetic inheritance of the thickest blood, coupled with agglutination from diet, and increased factors regarding stress.

So while all blood types are affected by stress to some extent, Type As, representing 40% of the world, are at the greatest risk, with ABs coming in a close second. It is for this reason we believe all type As should be vegetarian. In addition, nutritional supplements, such as ogliomeric proanthocyanidines, or super-antioxidants as well as vitamin E, resveratrol (plentiful in peanuts, grape juice, and red wine), which prevents clots from forming and appears to inhibit the oxidation of LDL cholesterol, a contributing factor in arterial degeneration, offer great protection from both heart disease and cancer.

In addition, Type As should incorporate green tea, soy beans, and/or tofu into their regulated diets. These provide numerous antioxidants, genistein, and estrogen that research has shown inhibits cancer.

BLOOD TYPE B

Type B blood was the third mutation through man's adaptation, after Types O and A. Individuals of this blood group share some characteristics of Types O and A, while some characteristics clearly set them apart from the other types. Although they represent a mix of the two previous blood types in some ways, there are some very notable exceptions.

Type B blood is not as thin as Type O blood, nor is it as thick as Type A blood. For the most part Type Bs can eat meat in moderation without great fear of developing heart disease. Although meat is not Type B's best food, it is not particularly harmful either. On the other hand, Type B individuals have the ability to eat and metabolize dairy products, which both Type O and Type A do not tolerate well at all.

In our research we found that the life spans of Type Bs mirrored the average life span of the United States. We found they were not immune to disease, but when they developed cancer or heart disease, they still tended to live longer than As or ABs who were afflicted. Also, we found individuals of Type B blood tended to contract diseases peculiar to their blood type, such as polio, lupus, and rare disorders such as Lou Gehrig's disease. Notwithstanding these very serious illnesses, most of the subjects managed to survive into their 70s, 80s, and some 90s.

It is believed improper foods, or the improper metabolism of specific foods, lower the immune system of Bs and makes them susceptible to autoimmune diseases. Some of these are life threatening, others just cause untold misery for life. The foods to avoid are noted in this book.

Another aspect of Type B individuals surprised us, in addition to longevity. Almost all the Bs we interviewed were highly intelligent. As a group they were extremely intelligent, deep-thinking individuals, who appeared to see the world from a slightly different viewpoint. Although they were obviously bright, they tended to be more introverted and disliked by the other blood types. Perhaps it is because they see things differently, and others don't agree with their thought processes, or perhaps the others harbor resentment because of their slightly different point of view. It wouldn't be the first time someone was disliked for his or her opinion. In spite of this fact, percentage-wise there are more B millionaires than of any other blood type.

As you will see by our statistics, Type B individuals average the second longest life span after Type Os, which win the longevity contest hands down. This is probably due to the fact that animal protein, which contains all those essential amino acids, is good food for Bs. Additionally, since Type Bs can eat a large variety of foods, they are able to acquire all or most of their essential vitamins, minerals and amino acids from food more easily than As and ABs.

Another striking fact we noticed was that Type B is the second most muscular, or has the genetics to be the second most muscular, next to Type O, who again win hands down. This is true with the exception of the A2 Type, many who build muscle just like Type O. In fact, in observing individual blood types engaged in body building the Os built muscle very quickly, followed by the Bs, then the ABs and finally the A1s who have a very difficult time.

As stated earlier, this is one reason why the overwhelming number of professional athletes are Type O, especially football, baseball, and basketball players, where size and strength count. While Bs build muscle easily, some gravitate to sports, perhaps as coaches and trainers, but the vast majority tends to pursue careers in medicine, law, science, and technology. They are professors and scholars, thinkers and dreamers, and represent 8% of the world population.

In interviewing numerous subjects of this group, most were healthy with some chronic medical problems. But we found the largest proportion of individuals who had suffered from polio, multiple sclerosis, and skin disorders such as psoriasis, eczema, fungus, and other skin conditions for which medical science appears to have difficulty treating or curing.

Another problem that kept popping up for Bs was foot problems of one kind or another. Numerous subjects had required foot surgery, or had problems with their feet which were very painful and made everyday walking difficult. However, most Bs were robust, healthy individuals who live long and productive lives.

The greatest numbers of Bs are from India. Again, if you will refer to Table 2, it indicates that Bs account for more than 40% of the population, while Os account for just over 30%. The reason for this is clear. Since India has not conquered typhoid, cholera, plague, and the other diseases that strike Os the hardest, many Os of the Indian culture have been struck down as they were in the middle ages.

BLOOD TYPE AB

Type AB is the only blood type that did not evolve in the same way as the other blood Types. While the other blood types have been around for thousands of years, Type AB has been in existence for only about 2,000 years. The genetic mystery of this blood type is complex. While the three other blood types evolved because of change of environment and food availability, Type AB did not.

It is believed Blood Type AB is the result of mixing Types A and B. However, since both A and B are dominant genes, genetically speaking, the offspring should have been A or B. But the question is "If A and B have been in existence for so long, what triggering event caused the mutation to AB?" And why does it happen in only rare instances? The answer, as far as we can determine, is not known, nor is the answer why there are not other mutations, which have produced other new blood types. Usually mutations come about to guarantee the survival of the species, and this might well be the reason for the AB mutation. Proponents of this theory would argue that this blood type is less susceptible to all of the diseases that strike Os the hardest, and as such, this is nature's way of evolving to insure the survival of the species.

What *is* known about AB is it is the only blood type with two dominant traits. That is, in terms of genetics, both Types A and B are dominant genes. To illustrate, if a parent of O Type blood mixes with a parent of A Type blood, the trait being dominant will prevail more times than the recessive trait O. The same holds true for B, which is also dominant over O. So when an A parent mixes with a B parent, the outcome genetically speaking should be either A or B, not AB. In any case, AB exists and represents about 2% of the population worldwide.

Since Type AB represents only 2% of the world's population, and is rare, it was difficult to find enough Type ABs for the study to yield precise results regarding longevity. However, from the statistics compiled we found some surprising consistencies, both positive and negative. On the negative side, ABs are susceptible to both A & B illnesses. So they are prone to cancer and heart disease by virtue of their A gene, and autoimmune diseases through the B gene. However, our research has not shown heart disease risks in ABs approaching that of As, perhaps because we were unable to locate more subjects, or they had died. We did find cancer rates approximately the same as As.

John F. Kennedy, who we know was AB, was exceptionally charismatic. He was known for many things.... keen mind, engaging personality, embodiment of youth, and overall charm made him one of our most beloved presidents. But along with this image was his preoccupation with the opposite sex. I think it's fair to say he was obsessed. Whether it was the times or his youthful and likable personality, the country was, and history may overlook his indiscretions. Only time will tell.

Historians have argued that JFK almost blew his career when he became obsessed with Marilyn Monroe. She too was obsessed with him. Marilyn Monroe was Type AB. We do not think this was a coincidence that the two were so fascinated with each other.

As you will see in the research, we found an overwhelming number of couples were married to an individual of the same blood type. Table 8 indicates 68%. Our research shows 14 ABs married to ABs. The statistical odds against that are in the billions. The same holds true for Bs and As and Os. The overwhelming data points clearly to the fact that couples are drawn to their mates through some blood type traits which are compatible with their own. This is the first and only study we know of that supports The Theory of Compatibility among humans according to blood type.

John F. Kennedy, Marilyn Monroe, and many other ABs possessed qualities quite unique as they all reached and influenced many people in a positive way, only to die sudden and tragic deaths. This is an interesting point, which we believe should be explored further.

Our research found most ABs likable, outgoing, gregarious, and intelligent people, at work and play. Many were professionals: doctors, lawyers, business owners, actors, as well as people in every walk of life.

Our research noticed a clear trend for women of this blood type to have many menstrual problems – excessive bleeding, clotting, cramping, irregular menstrual cycles – either leading to hysterectomies, or continued misery. The youngest in our sample was 27 years old.

Additionally, a large number of the women who experienced menstrual problems, also experienced migraine and other headaches. In my experience there is a strong possibility that the hormonal imbalance causing the menstrual difficulties may be partly responsible for the headaches. In either case, there is a clear pattern of hormonal imbalance that plagues this blood group more than others.

See: A Final Note (on page 257)

Another illness we saw over and over again in the AB blood type was bi-polar disorder (manic-depression). This too is believed to be an illness of chemical imbalance. This could be the result of two dominant genes attempting to exert their dominance, or perhaps because this blood type is a mutated merging of A and B, in the mutation lies strength and weakness.

Most of the ABs we encountered tended to be very self-confident and assertive individuals, who were able to achieve their goals in what appeared to others as seemingly effortless ways. Also, while most were outgoing and gregarious, the majority were loners, who preferred individual pursuits in medicine, dentistry, law, business, and acting.

In terms of muscular abilities, ABs were slightly more muscular than As, but less muscular than Bs. It was easier for an AB to build muscle than an A, but in some cases, ABs had as difficult a time building muscle as As. This, of course does not include the A2 Type, or "twisted A." Many of the ABs interviewed indicated that if they exercised regularly, they could become muscular, but soon after stopping lost muscle mass quickly. This would be consistent with the diverse A and B genes both exerting their dominant traits.

Eating properly for an AB requires guidelines similar to As, but with small amounts of animal protein. More than a little animal protein puts ABs in the same risk category as As for cancer and heart disease. ABs, like As, should acquire their vitamins, minerals and essential amino acids through plant and vegetable proteins, or suffer the consequences. Because eating properly is more difficult than it is for Os or Bs, who can do it much more easily in our culture, the life span of ABs appears to be about 70 years – longer than As generally, but not as long as Bs. The oldest Type AB we encountered was 83, and while he was not sick, he was not robust or physically active.

We believe this can be improved through proper diet and exercise. In addition to a multi-vitamin, the following recommendations are suggested: One 81.5-mg (baby) aspirin per day. Raw or dry-roasted red-skinned peanuts. If peanuts are a problem, try organic peanut butter or a 50- mg resveratrol supplement. One glass red wine per day, and one whey protein isolate supplement morning and evening, to insure all amino acids and protein requirements.

Lastly, ABs should incorporate green tea, soybeans, and/or tofu into their diets. These super foods contain antioxidants, genistein, and estrogen that research has shown inhibits cancer.

N ow that you understand the four blood types and how they evolved, it is important to focus on how and why diet is the culprit that kills many of us inadvertently, while sparing others. **Regardless of your blood type, the human life span can be increased as much as 20 years, especially in Type A and AB individuals, and to a lesser extent in Type O and B individuals.**

You are what you eat, but you should

"EAT WHAT YOU ARE"

This means each of us should eat the optimal diet compatible with our blood type. Doing this sounds easy enough, but in practice it is not.

For example, in the animal kingdom instinct is what drives animals to eat. Lions are meat eaters. Try and feed a lion carbohydrates such as fruits and vegetables, and you already know the result. Conversely, other animals are vegetarian, and by instinct, will not eat meat. This is no accident. Instinct is a protective mechanism for all animals. Awareness is the protective mechanism for humans. The problem is that humans are so domesticated that greater awareness is needed to drive their eating habits.

What we can learn from animals is they eat only what is instinctively good for them and as a result heart disease is virtually non-existent. While animals occasionally do develop cancer, statistically it occurs dramatically less often than in humans. Additionally, have you ever noticed that most animals of a given species all live to about the same age? Well, this is because of their uniform diets, driven by instinct that allow them to have life spans to the potential of their species. Another point to remember that is most animals that are not killed by predators die of old age, or what we call natural causes.

With humans it is just the opposite. Humans almost always die from one disease or another. As a result of our improper diets, our immune systems fail to operate properly and we become susceptible to one disease or another. Medical science has come a long way and has prolonged life for many. But as Ben Franklin once said, "An ounce of prevention is worth a pound of cure." These words of wisdom are still true today.

Yes, we have the ability to treat illness, and operate when necessary. But in many cases, much of what modern medicine does is treat the symptom or outward manifestation of the problem – not prevent the problem in the first place. It is not for us to place blame, as medicine is providing many wonderful cures, vaccines, and medications which are allowing people all over the world to live longer, more productive lives. However, we believe the emphasis currently is on the treatment, when more should be on prevention.

It all starts in our childhood. We grow up in families where we are given food our mothers and fathers believed was good for us, or tasted good. The fact that it tastes good is not an indication of whether the food is good for us. Our blood types were determined at the moment of conception, and although we may be able to change almost everything about ourselves, we cannot change our blood types, at least yet.

As discussed previously, each blood type has different characteristics that allow it to eat, digest, and assimilate the food best for that group. Since Os have been blessed with such strong stomach acid and respective enzymes, they are able to metabolize almost everything, even those foods not recommended for them. However, the Bs, As and ABs do not have this luxury, and accordingly must be more careful in their eating habits or suffer the consequences.

The Os are like sharks. Many are almost indestructible. They can eat tin cans, rubber tires, wash it down with hard liquor while smoking a cigarette, and not get indigestion. Of course, this is not true, but a dramatic exaggeration. Nevertheless, Type Os have the highest threshold for abuse than any other blood group, and in the final analysis, it is another reason they live longer.

Now let's get back to our eating habits and what happens when we eat food not compatible with our blood enzymes and stomach acid. Agglutination happens. What's that, you ask? Well, we humans have a process that takes place in our blood called agglutination.

Your body has antibodies that protect it from foreign invaders. Your immune system produces all kinds of antibodies to protect you and keep you safe from foreign substances. Each antibody is designed to attach itself to a foreign substance or antigen. When your body recognizes an intruder, it produces more antibodies to attack the invader. The antibody then attaches itself to the intruder and a "gluing" effect takes place. In this way the body can better dispose of these foreign invaders.

For example, if you eat a food not compatible with your blood type and stomach enzymes, the food is not broken down or digested properly, and the vitamins and minerals are not absorbed into your bloodstream to fuel and nourish your body. Your body reacts to the food just as it would any foreign substance. You might experience a stomach ache, gas, bloating, or even worse, vomiting or diarrhea. What happens is that antibodies glue themselves to the foreign invaders (improper food) and agglutination or "gluing" takes place in your blood.

Now if you happen to be Blood Type A, with already thick blood, your blood becomes even thicker. The thicker the blood, the slower it moves and the harder your heart must pump to push the blood through your arteries. This thick slow moving blood makes it easier for plaque to build up on your artery walls. Hence, high blood pressures, heart disease, or a cornucopia of other illnesses. You get the picture.

The human body is a wonderful and complex organism. It tries to handle everything you give it, but sometimes it cannot, or will not. The damage is greater or lesser, depending on how bad the food is for you and your particular body chemistry. If you are lucky, maybe this improper agglutination may result only in weight gain. The body does not use the food, so it just packs on extra pounds. You are not eating much, but you're gaining weight and don't know why. Well, the answer is improper metabolism of your food.

If you are Type A or AB and the meat you keep eating is not metabolizing, your bloodstream is now flooded with thick, sticky agglutinated blood, loaded with saturated animal fat, just looking for a nice spot to deposit itself. It doesn't take a genius IQ to see why As and ABs should not eat meat, and if they do, they die younger.

Now if O or B eat meat, their bodies metabolize it better, and the agglutination process does not take place, or if it does, it is very minor and not life threatening. Type Os, which usually completely metabolize meat and gain all the benefits from it (with the exception of pork), are at little or no risk. Further, since an O starts out with the thinnest blood, any agglutination that takes place does not do the damage experienced by the other blood types, or cause a life-threatening situation.

Take, for example, breads and white potatoes. If a Type O or Type A eats these foods, in most cases some agglutination takes place. However, since these foods contain little, if any fat, the body will not deposit the non-metabolized portion on the artery walls. It is more likely to store the unused food as fat. Hence, you gain weight. While this may be benevolent in the short run, eventually this excess fat may lead to diabetes, high blood pressure or other illnesses.

Any food containing saturated fat has the greatest potential for harm to the body in the long run, regardless of blood type. Saturated fat to Types A and AB is more dangerous in the short run because of the reasons stated previously. In the long run, even Types O and B, whose blood enzymes handle saturated fat better, are susceptible to the hazards. It just takes longer. So although Os and Bs are not particularly susceptible to heart disease and most forms of cancer, a continual regimen of saturated fat and/or incompatible foods will eventually produce the same result. It just appears the harmful effects take much longer in Os and Bs.

Saturated fats in the diet in any form will eventually undermine your health. Of the saturated fats, the most damaging come from animal protein. To eliminate this risk, acquire much of your protein, regardless of blood type, from sources that are fat-free, or free of animal saturated fat.

If some of this information is not familiar, refer to the Glossary in Appendix II for the pertinent terms on which all of this is based. In the final analysis, most of what needs to take place to avoid disease, boost immune function and maintain weight control – in short, to achieve the best result for your body – is all based on diet. **To succeed requires balancing proteins, carbohydrates, and fats in the proportions best for your body.**

As the body grows older, it stops producing certain hormones, it loses muscle mass, bones become more brittle, immune function decreases, and the body's intolerance of improper food begins to manifest itself in insidious ways.

But with proper diet, including nourishment from those foods and supplements specific to your needs, the chance of disease is greatly reduced. In fact, proper diet according to blood type, coupled with exercise, enables your immune system to be its strongest. A strong immune system can make the difference between a longer or shorter life span.

Since the body cannot repair itself without protein, protein is the key element in the equation for good health. We all must have protein; the form of that protein determines how long we will live. For individuals of Blood Types A and AB, animal protein from meat is unacceptable, with a few exceptions. For Bs, while meat is not particularly harmful in the short run, in the long run it contributes to heart disease and a host of other assorted ailments.

The body accesses body fat for fuel when it has burned its sugars and carbohydrates. The goal is to keep the body in an anabolic state for as many hours a day as possible. In this way the body always has the fuel it needs to rebuild and repair. Carbohydrates provide energy, but don't fulfill the body's need to build strong bones and boost immune function. In large amounts, carbohydrates place the body in a catabolic state, thereby affecting insulin levels and exposing the body to a host of dangerous and fatal ailments (i.e., diabetes and heart disease). (If some of these terms are not familiar, please refer to the glossary in Appendix II).

One way to insure that your body remains in an anabolic state is to add a protein supplement to your diet. One or two shakes a day will insure that your body remains in an anabolic state most of the day. It also allows you the ability to add only those beneficial fats and carbohydrates to your diet on a selective basis. We are of course referring to the polyunsaturated and monounsaturated fats.

By eliminating saturated fat from the diet and from protein sources, all blood types benefit by preventing the agglutination process and the heart disease, cancer, diabetes, and other ailments and diseases that ultimately can follow. By eating properly and following a sensible exercise program, each individual can maximize his or her potential life span.

Now let's try and be realistic. Many of you will not or cannot, because of lifestyle and scheduling conflicts, eat regularly and/or properly. In addition, even with the best of intentions many will not be able to exercise on a regular basis... or care to. However, you can still maintain the quality of life you desire by supplementing your diet with protein shakes (from powder sources) or health bars containing more protein than carbohydrate grams. At least in this way you are guaranteed to provide your body with all the essential protein your blood type requires.

CHAPTER IV

GENETICS AND ANTHROPOLOGY IN HUMANS

One of the most important abilities of humans is that of recognizing individual members of their own kind. It is an ability which we all take for granted; yet if one of us were unexpectedly asked how we did it, even an immediate, superficial answer would require a moment's thought.

Facial recognition is, of course, all important yet notoriously difficult to describe, especially when it is a matter of distinguishing between two or more members of one's own population or between persons of the same "race." One reason for this is that the mind, in interpreting the results of visual observation, pays considerable attention to facial "expression," which consists of subtle indications of the emotions of the person observed, brought about by slight contractions of the facial muscles. We have all seen a person alter in appearance, almost out of recognition, by the sudden removal of some source of worry, such as an unhappy personal relationship. Yet the shape of the face, and certainly the shape of the bones which form its main structure, have not changed at all. It is for this reason that the interpretations of the sensitive painter usually convey something different to us than the scientific descriptions of the anthropologist.

Yet, for scientific purposes we need to be able to describe the individual in unambiguous terms, which will mean the same to all readers.

Beyond the shape of the face as described above, the shape and size of the body and its parts also have descriptive importance. The color of eyes, hair and skin, and texture of hair are much easier to define than are subtle anatomical distinctions.

The characteristics just described are mainly inborn and hereditary rather than acquired, but some, especially body weight and the contours of the soft parts of the body, are mainly acquired and more dependent upon the state of nutrition.

In contrast to these visible characteristics, research during the present century shows a class of invisible ones, fixed by heredity in a known way at the moment of conception, immutable during the life of the individual, and observable by relatively simple scientific tests.

These are the "Blood Groups," to which have been added a large number of other chemical features of the blood in recent years. The most widely used of these sets of characteristics, recognized for almost 100 years now, is the system of ABO Blood Groups – Types A, B, AB, and O – to which all human beings belong, and which are familiar to all blood donors for transfusion. And discovered, it seems almost yesterday, are the HLA or histocompatibility groups, detected by blood tests but used to ascertain compatibility in the case of proposed grafts of kidneys and other organs.

In 1900, two events took place that rediscovered principles of the past, but up to this time were not seen as significant. Landsteiner in Austria discovered the human ABO Blood Groups, and Ehrlich and Morgenroth in Germany discovered similar phenomena in goats. The impetus came not from genetics or from human biology but from the techniques of bacteriology and the phenomenon of immunity to bacteria. When animals or human beings have been infected with certain bacteria, naturally or experimentally, their blood acquires the property of agglutinating preparations of the same bacteria. When serum from such blood is added to the uniform suspension of microscopic bacteria, it agglutinates or comes together in clearly visible clumps.

Blood is, of course, a suspension of microscopic red and white corpuscles in a fluid. The more numerous red corpuscles are, in fact, cells that have lost their nuclei; they are often referred to as "red cells." They consist of a membrane enclosing a solution of the red protein hemoglobin, which in the process of blood circulation serves to carry oxygen from the lungs to the tissues.

The white corpuscles, only about one one-thousandth as numerous, are true cells with a nucleus and cytoplasm. For the moment we shall be concerned solely with the red cells but shall return to the white cells later. The almost colorless fluid part of the circulating blood is known as "plasma." Plasma contains substances, which cause the blood to clot upon separation. When the clot has separated from the shed blood the remaining fluid, differing from plasma only in the absence of the clotting principles, is known as "serum."

Landsteiner laid the groundwork for we know today about blood transfusions. He found that when suspensions of red cells in weak salt solution (saline) from a number of individuals were tested separately by adding serum from other individuals, agglutination of the red cells took place in some but not in other cases. Landsteiner actually distinguished three types to which a fourth was very soon added.

The four blood types are now known as A, B, AB, and O, the symbol O indicating the absence, on the surface, of the red cells, of any of the blood group substances. The symbol A indicates the presence of a substance A on the cells, B the presence of a substance B, and AB the presence of both substances. For our purposes these substances are regarded as 'antigens', analogous to characteristic antigens present on the surface of bacteria.

It is the property of antigens that they combine with specific antibodies present in sera, the combination being demonstrated by a visible phenomenon such as agglutination. An antibody is named after the antigen with which it combines, preceded by the prefix 'anti-' the serum of a group A person contains the antibody anti-B; that of a group B person contains anti-A. The serum of a group O person contains both anti-A and anti-B, and that of a group AB person, neither. Thus the serum of any person contains as many kinds of antibodies as it can, subject to the limitation that the serum must not cause the agglutination of the subject's own red cells.

While this may seem complex to remember, the chart below illustrates this point that antigens generate antibodies.

TABLE 1

THE ABO BLOOD GROUPS: ANTIGENS AND ANTIBODIES

Blood Group	Blood Group Substances (Antigens in Red Cells)	Antibodies Present in Plasma (or serum)
O	NONE	ANTI-A ANTI-B
A	A	ANTI-B
B	B	ANTI-A
AB	A and B	NONE

The new discovery was presumably recognized at the outset as demonstrating a set of more or less permanent characteristics of individual human beings. At first, the blood groups were not seen as having any medical consequences, nor were they recognized as hereditary. Within a few years, however, they were shown to be indispensable indicators of compatibility between donors and recipients of blood given in transfusion. Blood transfusions had been attempted on many occasions during the previous 200 years in the treatment of hemorrhage or anemia, sometimes with success, but often followed by rather sudden and unexpected death, now recognized as being due to incompatibility. By this one discovery, transfusion was rendered almost completely safe.

D uring World War I a blood group researcher and physician, Ludwik Hirszfeld, and his wife, also a physician, served as army doctors at Salonika in northeastern Greece. This was an important communications center, a way station for a very large number of soldiers and refugees of great many nationalities. The Hirszfelds therefore decided to carry out blood group tests on large numbers of persons of as many races and nationalities as possible. The results of their tests are shown in Table 2.

It can be seen that when the same blood groups occurred in the populations tested, the percentages, or frequency of occurrence in each population, varied widely from one to another. The Hirszfelds tested soldiers of the many European nationalities of both the contesting armies, soldiers from many parts of Asia and Africa serving in the British and French colonial forces, as well as civilians from southeastern Europe. Apart from the Chinese and Japanese, and the indigenous peoples of Australia and America, in this one pioneer paper they established the main outlines of the world distribution of the ABO blood groups.

Moreover, unlike some of their successors, they realized the importance for reliable statistical results of testing large numbers, and to the extent possible, tested 500 members of each population group. Moreover, conscious of the anthropological importance of their results, they gave precise ethnic descriptions of their subjects, and of their places of origin. However, because their work did not fall into any recognized branch of science, and bore little relation to anything that had ever been published before, they had great difficulties in getting it published. There was a very long delay in acceptance by *The Lancet*, to which it was first offered, so it first appeared in the French journal *l'Anthropologie*.

TABLE 2

ABO BLOOD GROUPS AND POPULATIONS

Population	Number Tested	Blood Group Percentages			
		A	B	AB	O
United States	5,114	39.8	8.1	2.0	50.1
English	500	43.4	7.2	3.0	46.4
French	500	42.6	11.2	3.0	43.2
Italians	500	38.0	11.0	3.8	47.2
Germans	500	43.0	12.0	5.0	40.0
Serbs	500	41.8	16.2	4.6	38.0
Greeks	500	41.6	16.2	4.0	38.2
Bulgarians	500	40.6	14.2	6.2	39.0
Arabs	500	32.4	19.0	5.0	43.6
Turks	500	38.0	18.6	6.6	36.8
Russians	1000	31.2	21.8	6.3	40.7
Jews	500	33.0	23.2	5.0	38.8
Blacks	500	22.6	29.2	5.0	43.2
Indians (India)	1000	19.0	41.2	8.5	31.3

It was largely the discovery by the Hirszfelds of the varying frequencies of the blood groups in different populations and the elucidation of their mode of inheritance that led to the establishment of the science of population genetics, and we must now look at the blood groups from this standpoint.

Mendel in 1865 had established the importance of what are now called genes as the entities, which reappear, unchanged in generation after generation, in the process of reproduction. He himself was usually working with artificial populations of plants in which the frequencies of two genes were equal; that is to say the frequency of each gene was 50%. It is, however, implicit in his work that even if the gene frequencies are other than 50%, the initial frequencies will remain constant from generation to generation.

Let us now consider the specific example of the ABO blood groups in terms of the three genes – A, B, and O – the gene frequencies, as fractions (usually expressed as decimals) of unity, being given the symbols A, B, and O, respectively. In table 3 the sides of the square are each of value 1 (or 100 percent), and the area of the square thus has the value of 1 square unit. The values of the gene frequencies are shown along the edges of the square. We will regard vertical distances as the frequencies of the genes in the male reproductive cells and the horizontal distances as those of the genes in the female reproductive cells.

TABLE 3

	A	B	O
A	A	A-B AB	A-O
B	A-B AB	B	B-O
O	A-O	B-O	O

Diagram illustrating gene and gene frequencies. Each side of the square is assumed to be unity (100%), so that the total area is also unity. The divisions of the sides of the square represent the frequencies of the genes A, B, and O; the areas represent the genotypes resulting from all the possible pairings of these genes.

Not only is the study of natural selection of blood groups and other genetic characters therefore important for the anthropological interpretation of gene frequencies, but it has a very important future in medicine, helping us to predict and thus to guard against genetic tendencies to disease in individual patients. As such tendencies become better understood it may be found that a very large part of disease susceptibility is hereditary, but subject to control by suitable modification of the environment in the widest sense, **AND DIET**; the constant in the life of every human being and living organism.

CHAPTER VI

THE EVIDENCE OF
BLOOD GROUP ON LONGEVITY

The purpose of the following research was to establish a link between diet and disease. As the information began pouring in and it was sorted according to blood type, an amazing finding appeared over and over. The finding was that individuals of Blood Type A were dying at an alarmingly young age, from heart disease and cancer. Likewise, individuals who were living well into their 80s and 90s, some with disease but many without, were overwhelmingly Type O.

We were so amazed by these statistics we tried to find other sources of research wherein a correlation was made between blood type and longevity. We could find none.

Our sample includes more than 5,100 subjects, most of who were randomly chosen. Approximately 60 or 70 subjects were not chosen at random, as they were relatives and the data was easily obtainable (see Table 4).

Although most of our research subjects are American, foreigners are included in the sampling as well. Our research sample closely reflects the blood type percentages as they appear in the general population:

TABLE 4

BLOOD TYPE PERCENTAGES IN THE GENERAL POPULATION

	Total Number in Sample	Blood Type	Percentage of Whole
	2,433	O	47.7%
	1,842	A	36.1%
	621	B	12.0%
	218	AB	4.2%
TOTAL	5,114		100.0%

A representative sample of the study's subjects, living and deceased, is listed in Appendix I. The names have been changed to protect confidentiality. As Table 5 clearly indicates, you will see from the representative sample of each blood type, there are clear and convincing indications of a direct link between blood type and longevity. Although some would call this a coincidence, we believe **The Theory of Longevity** is correct. While this may be alarming or disheartening to many readers, and great news to others, it is expected that these numbers can and will be changed as more people learn how to adjust their diets and exercise in accordance with their blood types.

THE RESEARCH STUDY

Our research was conducted through surveys with people of each blood type. In addition to obtaining information about them, we asked information about their parents' or relatives' blood types, illnesses and cause of death, if known. For this reason, within the 5,114 samples, there are both living and deceased subjects.

We first determined the average age of the subjects within a blood type group (see chart below). The second figure is the subjects' average age at time of death. This figure represents the average life span within a blood group.

TABLE 5

LIFE SPAN TABLE AS PER BLOOD TYPE

Average Age of Sample	Blood Group	Average Age at Death
57.7	A	61.6
62.9	AB	69.5
67.6	B	78.2
78.5	0	86.7

The most significant finding resulting from Table 5 is that there is a direct link between blood type and longevity. At this time in the United States, individuals of blood type O live an average life span of approximately 25 years longer than individuals of blood type A. This gap is so significant it represents a priority that needs to be addressed NOW!

Another interesting aspect of the findings was when we averaged our data, taking into account the blood type, the average life span came out to 76.2 years, the same as reported by the United States government. However, if you are Type A or AB and think you will live to the average age of 76 years, you are clearly mistaken. So while the overall average life span is approximately 76, it is only because a very large part of the population (Type O) usually lives considerably longer, thereby skewing the figures for the entire population.

As Table 6 clearly indicates, heart disease and cancer are the major illnesses that strike all blood types. However, Table 7 shows that while everyone is susceptible, not all blood types are prone to contracting these illnesses at the same age.

TABLE 6
COMPOSITE DISEASE AND MORTALITY STATISTICS BY BLOOD TYPE

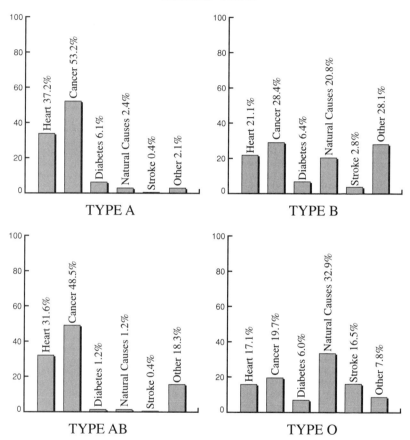

When you consider that heart disease and cancer are the number one and two killers, and that As and ABs have the highest heart disease and cancer rates, it is no surprise that the figures are slanted this way. We attribute these differences to diet. Since Blood Types A and AB do not tolerate meat well, it is predictable that in the United States, where meat is a staple, these two blood types average shorter lives.

TABLE 7

COMPOSITE GRAPHS PROFILING
MORTALITY STATISTICS BY DISEASE

Heart Disease (heart attack, heart failure, heart disease, etc.)

Age	Under 40		40-49		50-59		60-69		70-79		80-89		90-99		Over 100		Total
	M	F	M	F	M	F	M	F	M	F	M	F	M	F	M	F	
Type A	1.8	0.4	3.0		9.5	2.2	12.1	1.3	3.5	2.6		0.4	0.4				37.2%
Type B	0.9	0.9			0.9		0.9	0.9	4.6	5.6	1.8	3.7		0.9			21.1%
Type AB			0.4	0.4	0.4	0.4	12.7	0.4	10.6	6.3							31.6%
Type O								0.4	2.2	0.8	3.6	3.1	4.0	2.2		0.8	17.1%
TOTAL %	2.7	1.3	3.4	0.4	10.8	2.6	25.7	3.0	20.9	15.3	5.4	7.2	4.4	3.1		0.8	

Cancer

Age	Under 40		40-49		50-59		60-69		70-79		80-89		90-99		Over 100		Total
	M	F	M	F	M	F	M	F	M	F	M	F	M	F	M	F	
Type A	2.2	4.5	2.6	6.3	7.6	4.9	9.4	6.3	4.0	4.5	0.9	0.4					53.2%
Type B		1.8	0.9	2.8	0.9	0.9	4.6	1.8	4.6	3.7	3.7	1.8	0.9				28.4%
Type AB			4.2	10.6	4.2	2.1	14.8	4.2	6.3	2.1							48.5%
Type O				0.4	0.8	0.8	1.2	1.2	1.6	3.1	4.9	4.9	0.4	0.4			19.7%
TOTAL %	2.2	6.3	7.7	20.1	13.5	8.7	30.0	13.5	16.5	13.4	9.5	6.7	1.3	0.4			

Diabetes

Age	50-59		60-69		70-79		80-89		90-99		Over 100		Total
	M	F	M	F	M	F	M	F	M	F	M	F	
Type A		0.9		2.2	1.7	1.3							6.1%
Type B					2.8		1.8	1.8					6.4%
Type AB			0.8	0.4									1.2%
Type O					0.4	2.2	1.2	2.2					6.0%
TOTAL %		0.9	0.8	2.6	4.9	3.5	3.0	4.1					

Natural Causes

Age	50-59		60-69		70-79		80-89		90-99		Over 100		Total
	M	F	M	F	M	F	M	F	M	F	M	F	
Type A			0.4	0.4		0.8	0.4	0.4					2.4%
Type B					0.4		4.6	5.6	5.6	4.6			20.8%
Type AB					0.4		0.4	0.4					1.2%
Type O						0.4	4.9	3.1	10.3	9.4	3.6	1.2	32.9%
TOTAL %			0.4	0.4	0.8	1.2	10.3	9.5	15.9	14.0	3.6	1.2	

It should be noted all blood types are susceptible to any disease or illness. What is significant is the fact not all blood types seem to be susceptible at the same stage in life.

As indicated above, all blood types died from heart disease and cancer, the number one and two killers in this country. However, As and ABs died at much younger ages from these diseases than Bs and Os. In fact, if you take all diseases, the individuals of Blood Type O seemed to contract life-threatening diseases at a later stage than the other three blood types. For example, Type Os did not begin showing evidence of heart disease until well into their 60s and 70s, while Type As showed signs of heart disease as early as their 30s and 40s. We are sure individuals of Blood Type O experience heart disease before their 60s, but our research found only a few, and all were doing well with few restrictions.

Men of Blood Types A and AB, from their 40s through their 60s, showed a significantly higher death rate from heart attack and heart disease than their female counterparts. We attributed this to the hormonal protection women benefit through menopause, after which our research showed the Type A women had approximately the same risk for heart disease as the Type A men in their later years.

Although cancer did show beginnings in all blood types as early as the 30s and 40s, the mortality rates from cancer were much higher at younger ages for the Type As and ABs, who more frequently died in their 40s, 50s and 60s. Type Os died more often in their 70s and 80s from cancer.

As noted in Table 7, the Type Bs had the highest percentage of "other" illnesses and diseases (28.1%) – many of which are autoimmune diseases like Lou Gehrig's disease, lupus, cerebral palsy, multiple sclerosis, rheumatoid arthritis, etc. – that they died from. Because of this reason, they are a much more difficult blood type to classify. However, the majority of Type Bs "dodged" the illness bullet, and were remarkably healthy, as evidenced by their second longest life span, after Type O.

It also is interesting to note that more Type Os died of natural causes in their 80s, 90s, and 100s, than any other blood type group. A substantial number died in later years of stroke, which we attribute to the thinner blood that does not clot well after an artery in the brain ruptures. Type Bs showed some significant numbers dying of natural causes in their 80s and 90s, while a very small percentage of Type As and ABs died of natural causes.

Since Types A, AB, and B make up approximately 50% of the population worldwide, it is imperative that we address health and medical issues according to blood type. More research needs to be done so that our entire society will benefit by living healthier, more productive and longer lives.

If you are Blood Type O, you may not feel this information is urgent to know, since you will probably live longer and probably have parents and relatives who lived long lives. However, the genetic chart (Table 3) on page 72 indicates, just because you may be Blood Type O does not mean your children, spouse, or other relatives will be. In fact, statistically almost all families have more than one blood type within the family unit. We all carry a dominant and recessive gene, with the exception of an AB, who carry two dominant genes. We came across situations where one parent was AB, the other O. This happens frequently because the AB cannot find another AB, and consequently gets along well with Type O. The AB father passed the B dominant gene to his first daughter, the A dominant gene to his son, giving rise to an A child and a B child, resulting in four family members with four different blood types. This is not common, but does exist. Also, our research indicated that the AB parent gave off the B gene more often than the A gene. The reasons for this are not yet known.

Every time we read the results of the latest survey to test a drug, herb, or diet, usually the results are mixed and inconclusive. We believe this is attributable to the fact that all of these drugs, herbs, or diets will help some but not others, and the results will almost always be mixed. When studies are done within a blood type, the results will be more accurate than the present system of using a cross section of the population.

Two examples are aspirin and vitamin E. We believe aspirin and vitamin E are life savers and miracle substances, on a prophylactic basis, for individuals of Blood Types A and AB. This is because aspirin and vitamin E both thin the blood and protect against heart disease and some cancers. Since As and ABs have thicker blood than O and B, this thinning effect tends to prevent clots from forming. If a clot does form, aspirin and vitamin E may help to dissolve it or lessen the harmful effects. Conversely, we would not recommend these substances for Blood Types B and O because they would tend to make their blood too thin, which could cause excess bleeding and other related problems. **Please consult your own physician for specific advice regarding aspirin and vitamin E.**

It is interesting to note that Japan – a country consisting of predominately Type As – holds the record for the longest life span of any country in the world: 78 for men, 83 for women. The reason for this phenomenon is the Japanese eat in accordance with their blood type. For centuries, their staple diet has been fish, rice, soy products and green tea. This diet, which consistently promotes their good health, is the reason why Type A Japanese live much longer than their counterpart Type A Americans.

As far as our research goes it appears the Japanese are the only people who for centuries have married, hired, eaten, and incorporated many of the blood type characteristics into their daily lives. When you consider that the Japanese, who are predominantly Type A, have very low heart disease and the American As have the highest, we conclude it is their highly beneficial diet, low in saturated fats and high in monounsaturated (good fat) from fish, that makes the difference.

As the Japanese become more Americanized and as the consumption of beef increases in Japan, as it has for several years, the life span of the Japanese will begin to fall in direct proportion to their abandonment of their traditional diet in favor of a more westernized diet.

CONCLUSIONS

We believe all blood types should theoretically live approximately the same life spans.

- We believe that if individuals of Blood Types A and AB eat and exercise in accordance with the guidelines of this book, they can increase their life expectancy as much as 20 years.*

- We also believe that if individuals of Blood Type B eat and exercise in accordance with the guidelines of this book, they can increase their life expectancy as much as 8 to 15 years.*

- We further believe that if individuals of Blood Type O eat and exercise in accordance with the guidelines of this book, they can increase their life expectancy as much as 5 to 10 years.*

*These estimates depend on how early in life one changes lifestyle and his or her current medical condition at the time.

By implementing these changes in our daily lives all people will live longer, healthier, and productive lives. No longer will it be guesswork as to what to eat and what not to eat. It will be the understanding that as humans of different blood types we have specific individual needs that allow us to be our best. The answer has always been within our grasp.

THE ANSWER IS IN YOUR BLOODTYPE.

When we first began this research, the link we were looking for involved how diet and disease are interrelated. After further analysis, we found an overwhelming number of couples share the same blood type.

The first striking realization of this came when we learned one of our researchers had the rarest blood type. It made little difference to him he was AB. When he found out that AB represents 2% of the world's population, it still was no big deal. But when we tested his mate and fellow researcher, and she too was AB, we were shocked, surprised, and gratified all at the same time. We had two more blood tests to confirm the results, and sure enough, they were the same.

Okay, that could be a coincidence. But then we found another man who was AB, and we found out his wife was also AB, we were truly shocked and amazed. We found another couple, from India, and they too were AB. When we found the third, fourth and fifth couples all AB and married to ABs, we knew something else was going on that needed to be explored further.

We decided that perhaps it would be a good idea to start checking couples for blood type, unrelated to disease, and what we found was extremely interesting. Slowly but surely a pattern started to emerge showing a clear and overwhelming majority of couples with the same blood type.

The first and easiest place to inquire is your family. As it turned out one of our researchers had 12 cousins, all Blood Type B. When we checked their spouses, every one was married to another B. Now B only represents 8% of the population, so the chances of all of them marrying Bs was slim, statistically speaking. But it was true. Then we found more Bs married to Bs. The chance of this happening over and over again was astronomical.

My mate has three sisters, blood Type A, all married to As. As we continued to check couples, the percentage of couples of the same blood type exceeded 65%. We next looked at the couples with different blood types, and other patterns emerged. The following are the results:

TABLE 8

COMPATIBILITY TABLE

Total number of couples in study	721
Percentage of same bloodtype marriages or relationships	68%
Percentage of different bloodtype marriages or relationships	32%
Least compatible bloodtypes	A and B

We found an overwhelming number of couples married to spouses of the same blood type, and of those, we found the divorce rate lower than in individuals of different blood types. This doesn't mean that parties of the same blood type don't get divorced, but there is a greater likelihood spouses of the same blood type have more in common, and have a better chance of staying together than the inverse. This might account for so many divorces.

In light of this seemingly unusual pairing of individuals of the same blood type, we have drawn general conclusions, which are not etched in stone. There are always exceptions to every rule, and we expect this chapter will be most controversial. However, this data was collected and collated with no prior expectation in mind. It wasn't until some very real patterns began to emerge that we felt compelled to point them out. Perhaps as a result of this publication, more research will be done that will shed more light on this subject.

The conclusions and patterns of compatibility are as follows:

All blood types get along with their same blood type. The overwhelming number of subjects in the sample tests were married to mates within their blood type group. More type Os were married to Os, and As married to As, and so on.

We also found that although this was the most common combination of couples, there seemed to be a pattern that ran along bloodlines similar to the way people can give and receive blood.

Example:

- **Blood Type O is the universal donor. Blood Type O appears to get along best with another O, but is compatible with individuals of all other blood types.**

- **Blood Type AB is the universal receiver. Blood Type AB appears to get along best with another AB, but is compatible with individuals of all other blood types.**

- **Blood Type A can only receive blood only from another Blood Type A or O. Blood Type As get along best with another A, then O, but does not get along well with Blood Type B.**

- **Blood Type B can only receive blood only from another Blood Type B or O. Blood Type Bs get along best with another B, then O, but do not get along well with Blood Type A.**

Our research showed that of those individuals not the same type, more As and ABs were together, as were Bs and Os, more times than not. Perhaps the meat eaters (Types B and O) and non-meat eaters (Types A and AB) have something in common that attracts them.

We found that couples of Blood Types A and B, respectively, had more difficult relationships with each other and a higher divorce rate than other blood types. In other words, their compatibility factor was lower than parties of the same blood type, or more compatible blood types listed above.

The research on this matter is only a by-product of the basic research originally done. There is reason to believe although humans appear to have lost most of their instinctual responses because of modern technology, changes in environment, and a host of other reasons, there is a sixth sense which we don't fully understand and which guides us in our daily lives.

It may influence why we are drawn to certain individuals who on the surface do not seem suited to us. Or, why people with self-destructive natures are drawn to individuals who are bad for them. In either case, we believe more research needs to be done in this area.

SEXUAL COMPATIBILITY

The results in this section are based on data provided by 320 couples who agreed to discuss the most intimate details regarding their sex lives with their spouses. Prior to this research, it would have never occurred to us there might be a link between blood type and sexual compatibility. But in light of the findings of similarities in other areas, it is now not surprising there is a link between partners and their sexual preferences. The sample consisted of the following:

Total Number of Couples in Survey: **320**

Total Number of Couples with Same Blood Type: **218**

Percentage of Couples with Same Blood Type: **68%**

TABLE 9

SEXUAL COMPATIBILITY TABLE

		Percentage
Total Number of Couples Both of Type O	114	35.6%
Total Number of Couples Both of Type A	99	30.9%
Total Number of Couples Both of Type B	18	5.7%
Total Number of Couples Both of Type AB	7	2.1%
Total Number of Couples of Type A or AB	18	5.7%
Total Number of Couples of Type O or B	21	6.6%
Total Number of Balance of Couples	43	13.4%

Table 9 clearly shows many couples share the same blood type. Is this a coincidence? We think not. When you look at the ABs and Bs who make up the smallest percentages of the population, and when you calculate the possibilities of these groups having such a high incidence of compatibility, it would seem extremely unlikely according to the law of averages. The mere fact that we found so many type B couples, AB couples, etc. is beyond the realm of normal probability.

We believe something accounts for this high incidence of compatibility according to blood type. The logical conclusion is that individuals of a given blood type are inherently drawn to other individuals of the same blood type. Perhaps it is instinct or some factor of compatibility at play we don't fully understand. In either case, further research is needed to understand this phenomenon.

Our survey asked more than 750 individuals one additional question, which 320 agreed to answer.

QUESTION: Which best describes your sex life?

Vigorous

Moderate

Slow & easy

THE RESULTS ARE ON TABLES 10 & 11:

TABLE 10

SEXUAL PREFERENCES BY BLOOD TYPE

14 people of Blood Type O responded as follows:	Percentage
78 answered *Vigorous*	68.4%
21 answered *Moderate*	18.4%
15 answered *Slow & Easy*	13.2%
68 people of Blood Type B responded as follows:	Percentage
23 answered *Vigorous*	33.8%
35 answered *Moderate*	51.5%
10 answered *Slow & Easy*	14.7%
110 people of Blood Type A responded as follows:	Percentage
20 answered *Vigorous*	18.2%
41 answered *Moderate*	37.3%
49 answered *Slow & Easy*	44.5%
8 people of Blood Type AB responded as follows:	Percentage
4 answered *Vigorous*	14.3%
10 answered *Moderate*	35.7%
14 answered *Slow & Easy*	50.0%

TABLE 11

QUICK COMPARISON OF SEXUAL PREFERENCES

	Vigorous	Moderate	Slow & Easy
Blood Type O	68.4%	18.4%	13.2%
Blood Type B	33.8%	51.5%	14.7%
Blood Type A	18.2%	37.3%	44.5%
Blood Type AB	14.3%	35.7%	50.0%

CONCLUSIONS

The pattern of As and ABs preferring slow and easy sex over vigorous and moderate could be a coincidence, but we don't think so. Considering Blood Types A and AB prefer less vigorous forms of exercise such as walking, bicycling, golf, yoga and tai chi, a logical conclusion is that their sexual preferences would mirror their exercise patterns, or vice versa.

The pattern of Bs and Os preferring physically vigorous and moderate sex could also be a coincidence. But again, we don't think so. Considering that their exercise profiles show they prefer more vigorous forms of exercise such as aerobics, jogging, and weight training, a logical conclusion could be drawn that their sexual preferences would mirror their exercise pattern, or vice versa.

WORK COMPATIBILITY

We also examined how one's blood type may affect career choice. Since it was difficult to describe the compatibility of blood type with numerous career fields, we chose police work and firefighters because inherent in these career choices are certain physical challenges. Our goal was to see if a pattern could be found. The findings are as follows:

Number of Subjects in Sample: **356**

TABLE 12

WORK COMPATIBILITY STATISTICS

Number of subjects with Blood Type O:	279	79%
Number of A1 subjects:	8	2%
Number of A2 subjects:	49	14%
Number of subjects with Blood Type B:	18	5%
Number of subjects with Blood Type AB:	2	.005%

CONCLUSION

An overwhelming number of police officers were Blood Types O and A2s. Nearly all the As were determined to be A2 type. Very few were Types B and AB. This finding runs parallel to those concerning exercise and sexual preferences. Types O and A2 are probably drawn to police work because it is perceived as physically demanding work. A1s and ABs tend to shy away from work that is more physically demanding, perhaps because they don't have the muscle mass, or because it is inconsistent with their overall personality profile.

A small sample of 388 firefighters also was tested, but we did not feel this constituted a large enough group to be representative. However, even among the limited sample, the results were approximately the same as the police sample. We think more research in this area is needed in order to form a sound conclusion.

CHAPTER VIII

EXERCISE

E xercise is another component of good health. This chapter examines exercise and the benefits it bestows on the body.

We think it is fair to say most people hate to exercise. The reasons not to exercise number in the thousands, and we're probably missing some. But the point is, with the exception of the hard core few, the rest of us dislike exercise. Let's face it, after a long day's work, who wants to exercise? We want to relax, kick back, and enjoy what little time we have for other activities.

Unfortunately, as much as we hate to do it, exercise is a necessary requirement of good health for everyone, of every blood type. Now we all know people who have lived to a ripe old age, did no exercise, smoked like a chimney, and drank to excess. They were probably Type Os, and if anyone can get away with it, it is the Os, but we shouldn't count on it.

The body requires exercise; otherwise it responds as any other machine that isn't used. It rusts, gets stiff, begins to malfunction and finally breaks down. Exercise keeps the joints oiled, the machinery working properly, the hormones pumping, and in conjunction with the proper diet, keeps us younger for a longer period of time. If you were to compare your body to a car, and you only ran the car only one day a week, how well do you think it would run?

Your body is the machinery you were given for a lifetime. None of us have any control over the unforeseen, but we all have control over what we choose to put in our bodies. So if you put the wrong fuel in your car and let it sit idle, the lack of use is followed by a reduction of function. Now that we all understand the basics, let's see what exercise does for the body in conjunction with the proper diet and supplements.

Exercise strengthens bones, which make up your skeleton. The infrastructure around which the muscles, ligaments, cartilage, and skin operate must be strong. Exercise also strengthens bone density, prevents or minimizes the risks of osteoporosis, and allows individuals to be more vigorous in every way.

Exercise fortifies the muscles, ligaments, and cartilage by increasing blood flow to these and other vital organs. This blood flow, or river of life, that traverses the human body, cleanses and delivers food and oxygen to every living cell. This river of blood not only nourishes the entire body with vitamins, minerals, and nutrients but also bathes every organ while removing waste from the human environment.

Exercise requires more blood flow to provide additional oxygen to the body. Blood is tissue in liquid form. Separate it and you have three distinct layers – plasma, white blood cells, and red blood cells. The red cells, numbering between 20 and 30 trillion, make up approximately 45% of the blood's volume, depending on the urgency of the body's tasks. These plump red cells carry oxygen to the cells, while removing the carbon dioxide to be disposed as waste. Red blood cells consist primarily of water and **red protein** called hemoglobin. **It is the power of this protein that gives the red blood cell its vast oxygen-carrying capacity.**

Constructed from more than 10,000 atoms, a hemoglobin molecule consists of four elaborately entwined strands of **amino acids** called globin. In the middle of each strand is the heme, a disk of carbon, hydrogen, and nitrogen atoms with a single iron atom wedged in the center. The iron atom in heme acts as a magnet, attracting oxygen, then clinging to it tightly.

When oxygen is plentiful, as in the lungs, iron exercises its full powers, vacuuming up oxygen molecules. Conversely, when the oxygen supply is low, the body does not function at full potential and you feel sluggish and lazy. So in reality exercise provides the body with more energy, not less, as many people think.

Exercise raises your HDL, your "good cholesterol." Remember, there is "good" and "bad" cholesterol. The bad is LDL. When you exercise your HDL cholesterol goes up, and this in turn helps reduce your LDL cholesterol and your blood lipids or triglycerides. The net result is a better HDL/cholesterol ratio, which in turn reduces the risk of heart disease, diabetes, stroke, and a host of other potential medical ailments.

Exercise lowers blood pressure. This happens for many reasons. First, as you increase your blood flow and oxygen, your blood vessels dilate to accommodate the additional flow required to supply the body's requirements. Next, as your HDL goes up and LDL goes down, there is a cleansing effect on your blood vessels whereby any buildup of plaque or saturated fat is carried away, thereby allowing the heart to pump blood through the arteries more efficiently.

Exercise increases your metabolism. Your metabolism is the rate at which your body burns food and converts it to energy. If you live a sedentary lifestyle, rarely doing any exercise, your body metabolism is slowed and you require less food to fuel it. But if you exercise regularly, your body metabolism will speed up and require more food (fuel). The question might be asked, why should I try to speed up my metabolism, thus requiring more food? There are a number of reasons.

First, the less food you eat, the less chance you have to acquire the vitamins, minerals, and amino acids necessary to complete nutrition. Conversely, the more you eat the better chance your body has to acquire all of the above for good health. **So if you don't or can't eat right, you should at least supplement your body several times a day with a protein shake which contains all the essential amino acids your body requires, and/or vitamin supplementation.**

Second, a slow metabolism will allow foods to travel through your body at a slower rate. Once your body has derived what it can from food, it expels the waste products. The longer this unused portion of your food remains in your body the greater potential for harm, such as colon cancer. A faster metabolism speeds up the process and removes potential carcinogens from your system more quickly.

Exercise increases your body level of human growth hormone, also known as HGH. What is HGH and why is it important? HGH is a hormone excreted by the pituitary gland. Up to age 21 the body secretes this hormone in regular doses, and as such the body ages very little. After age 21 the body slowly secretes less and less of this anti aging hormone, and eventually by age 50 or 60 there is little if any secreted. The result is that about 1/3 of the aging population does not secrete HGH because they live a sedentary lifestyle.

This hormone that is secreted by the pituitary gland through exercise is the closest thing to an anti-aging bullet we have in nature. Studies have proven that moderate exercise extends your life. In fact, a famous study at Harvard University looked at alumni between the ages of thirty-five and seventy-five, and found that men who did moderate to vigorous exercise, such as tennis, swimming, jogging, or brisk walking, lowered their overall death rates by 25 to 33 percent, and reduced their risk of cardiovascular disease by an astounding 41 percent, when compared to the inactive alumni.

Exercise sends a wake-up call to your pituitary to secrete higher levels of growth hormone. And the superstar exercise to send your growth hormone levels surging is weight-resistance training. Lifting weights can do things for your body that you never dreamed possible, and you're never too old to start.

In the future you will hear more and more about HGH because in conjunction with the proper foods for your blood type, there does not exist a more potent one two punch for reversing the effects of aging.

You get the idea. The human body is an intricate instrument, unlike anything before it, and the most highly specialized form of life that has ever inhabited on this planet. But to keep the body in its peak form requires you to feed it only those foods that provide the blood with what your body really needs, and exercise it to keep all the parts moving properly. Unnecessary or harmful foods that agglutinate the blood, combined with a lack of exercise, will turn your blood to sludge, your performance to failure, depress your immune system, and decrease your potential maximum life span.

So we ask the question;
What exercise is best for me?

This varies from person to person, but whatever form of exercise you choose, it should be something you like and will stick with for an extended period of time. There is no use attempting exercise that is incompatible with your personality, or will lead to burnout. Exercise may seem easy, but as you already know, very few people stick to an exercise program, unless they truly like or believe in it.

But as just stated above, the single most beneficial exercise, for those who do not have an impediment, is weight-resistance training. It provides weight loss, builds muscle, strengthens the immune system, lowers blood pressure and cholesterol, and reverses the effects of aging. It does not require using heavy weights, or the effort which competitive bodybuilders put into the sport. For people in their 70's 80's and 90's the studies show immense benefits through weight resistance training.

Which brings us to the next step – commitment. Without a commitment on your part to be healthier and to follow the rules of your body's requirements, you are just fooling yourself. Before you undertake a regular exercise program, first consult with your doctor to make sure there are no impediments to your taking on the program. After you have been given a clean bill of health, make the necessary commitment and follow through. Remember, the more you put into this effort, the more you will realize out of it.

Because we believe weight resistance training is so beneficial, let's look at one type of resistance training you may not be familiar with.

CIRCUIT TRAINING

There are various methods of resistance or weight training. A common misconception that has been accepted through the years regarding resistance training, particularly lifting weights, is that muscles will hypertrophy or grow to extreme sizes and therefore cause a person to become 'muscle bound.' The truth of the matter is that the development of lean muscle mass, through resistance training, is a very welcomed condition to be acquired and for many obvious reasons. One important benefit received when lean muscle is added to one's body composition is that muscle tissue serves as a mechanism by which the body can burn additional calories throughout the day.

Another misconception held by many is that this method of exercising is simply anaerobic and does nothing to improve or stimulate the cardiovascular system. Resistance training does produce lean muscle mass and is anaerobic, but also promotes or stimulates heightened cardiovascular function while toning and reshaping muscle. This is accomplished when 'circuit training' is implemented as the methodology of exercise.

Circuit training is a method of toning and strengthening muscle and stimulating the cardiovascular system while not placing the emphasis on muscle overloading or maximum muscle development, as do other types of resistance training. Rather, maintaining an elevated training heart rate for a longer period of time, which then allows the body to draw from fat as its primary source of fuel. This concept of exercise is ideal for all blood types because it is not so intense that a Blood Type AB would be overly stimulated but by the same token a Blood Type O could get stimulated.

Circuit training is ideal for those who are particularly interested in maintaining a level of cardiovascular and musculoskeletal fitness, reduced inches and body fat, and to maintain lean muscle mass. Circuit training is performed by using a variety of stations on a multi-station exercise machine, the use of dumbells, or flex chords, such as the Rock and Roller Total Fitness Bar. The exerciser completes 30 seconds of exercise followed by a 15-30 second rest interval. If preferred, a specific amount of repetitions may be used (15-20), instead of time intervals. Typically, the exerciser will continue through all exercises or exercise stations, which completes a full circuit. Dependent upon the individual's fitness condition, two or more circuits may be performed. It is important to stay within the prescribed training heart-rate zone.

CIRCUIT TRAINING PRIMER

The following is a typical example of how circuit training is performed. The sequence, variety of exercise selection, method of exercise, (free weights or machines) and weight is based upon the physical condition of each individual.

Perform up to 20 repetitions per exercise in 30 seconds. Then rest for 30 seconds. Move to the next exercise and repeat. Continue until all the exercises listed in your program are completed. This completes one entire circuit with a 30 seconds on, and 30 seconds off tempo. Remember to adjust the amount of weight per exercise so that the 20th repetition is challenging.

Note: Before you attempt the outlined training or any exercise program, always consult your physician. Now let's look at a typical circuit training set of exercises.

EXAMPLE: 1 complete circuit with the use of dumbbells.

(1) Bench Press	**(6) Crunches**
(2) Lateral Rises	**(7) Triceps Extensions**
(3) Deep Knee Bends	**(8) Calf Raises**
(4) Biceps Curls	**(9) Hip Flexors**
(5) 1-Arm Rows	**(10) Lunges**

A second and third circuit may be added as the individual becomes more physically fit.

This method of exercise is very effective for improving the cardiovascular system, firming, toning and strengthening muscles while using body fat for energy.

For best results, a program designed according to the physical condition and goal of the individual with a method of monitoring progress is recommended.

Now, for those who cannot or choose not to use resistance training, let's look at some other exercise options, and the benefit of some of the research we have done in this area.

We have found that individuals of Types O, B, and A2 blood appear to like and respond well to intense physical exercise. This would include running, (jogging), aerobics, weight training, stair climbing, and any other physically demanding activity. Individuals of Types A and AB tend to gravitate to exercise that is less strenuous, such as walking, treadmill, golf, dancing, exercise bike, and stretching exercises such as yoga. All of the above exercises will raise your HGH levels and extend your life.

However, there are no hard and fast rules on this matter. People tend to gravitate to activities that make them feel good and what they like, regardless of how strenuous. I have seen A1s and ABs working out in the gym doing weight training, and Os and Bs doing walking and yoga. It is just a personal preference. The main thing is to get regular exercise, 20 to 60 minutes, three times a week, for all of the reasons previously stated.

Remember that after you exercise, work a hard stressful day, or exert yourself in any way, the body needs protein to repair itself. It is the protein – not the carbohydrates or fat – that repairs the muscles, ligaments, cartilage. For best results you should provide your body with the best sources of protein available consistent with your blood type. Protein is evaluated by the biological value or BCAA's (branch chain amino acids) provided.

This is a scientifically derived method of measuring the amount of nitrogen – retention supplied by a protein source. It is the function of a protein's amino acid content, digestibility and utilization, and is based on human experiments, not rat experiments like other outdated forms of measurements. The following are the scientifically rated protein sources in terms of the biological value provided to the body, which then maintains growth, repair and build muscle, increase body metabolism, create an anabolic over catabolic cycle, monitor water balance, and strengthen immune function in the body.

TABLE 13

RANKING OF PROTEIN SOURCES

1. Personal Protein™ *(Whey Protein Isolate)*		*159*
2. Regular Whey		104
3. Whole Egg		100
4. Egg White (albumin)		96
5. Whole Milk		91
6. Beef		80
7. Casein-Milk Protein		77
8. Soy		74
9. Wheat		54
10. Beans		49

Whey protein isolate is rated so highly by the medical profession that it is used to treat individuals whose immune systems are impaired or compromised and by elevating deficient levels of glutathione, an extremely important antioxidant involved in the maintenance of functional and structural integrity of muscular tissue undergoing oxidative damage during exercise and aging.

Now we know many of you, especially individuals of Type O and B blood would prefer to eat beef, rather than take a protein supplement. So for those who want the comparison, the following chart rates Personal Protein against your favorite cut of beef. This is not to suggest that you should give up that delicious cut of beef, but an accurate comparison of the two will keep this issue in perspective. Nutritional values based on an 8-ounce portion:

TABLE 14
PERSONAL PROTEIN VS. BEEF

Protein Source	Fat Grams	Calories	Calories from Fat	Protein	Cholesterol
Top Round	22.5	416	49%	46 grams	144 mg
Sirloin	36.7	512	65%	43 grams	152 mg
Prime Rib	74.6	944	71%	35 grams	168 mg
New York Strip	40.6	544	67%	42 grams	152 mg
Porterhouse	49.2	616	72%	40 grams	152 mg
T-Bone	49.5	616	72%	40 grams	152 mg
Rib-Eye	39.7	616	58%	40 grams	152 mg
London Broil	24.1	408	53%	45 grams	120 mg
Delmonico	49.0	584	75%	40 grams	152 mg
Filet Mignon	52.0	656	71%	40 grams	160 mg
Personal Protein (2 1/2 Scoops)	0	187.5	0%	45 grams	7.5 mg

While beef is very beneficial for Type O and neutral for B, we still believe when you look at the data comparing the sources of protein, you will come to the same conclusion we have. Protein supplements are an essential part of everyone's diet, and should be used in conjunction with other beneficial foods for your blood type.

CONCLUSION

Proper diet and regular exercise are the keys to staying younger longer, building a stronger immune system, and in general, are your best bet to avoid disease and maintain vitality. Together, they offer the best strategy to enable the body to stay strong, youthful, and healthy. It isn't magic, but it is real, and it works.

You have seen the statistics on longevity. You have been given the fundamentals of the proper diet, based upon your blood type. You have more information at your disposal than at any time in history to help you extend life as much as 20 years or longer, depending on when you start, and your ability to stay the course. It is now up to you to take these fundamentals and apply them to yourself. We believe if you follow the universal rules, as outlined in your genetics, it will be the best investment you will ever make.

No one can do this for you. It requires commitment, determination, and discipline. But what else are you doing with your life that is more important than your health? If for no other reason, we urge you to make the commitment for 30 days and see how you feel, and how your body reacts. We believe you will be surprised and pleased. You can procrastinate, deny, or ignore the information provided in this book, but for the overwhelming number of individuals, it is the best way to insure your future health and well-being.

You may not see the urgency of starting this program right away. You may be a teenager or a middle-aged individual in excellent health. But eventually the end must come for us all. Most people want to see their children grow and prosper, and to reap the rewards of all of their endeavors. To see one's life cut down in its prime is a tragedy that now may be prevented.

Most people think they will live the usual life span plus a few years. Very few think they will be the one to have the fatal heart attack, cancer, or unexpected illness. But the statistics are there, and cannot be ignored without consequences. Although we cannot change what has transpired, we do have the ability to change the future.

In the final analysis, exercise and the proper diet are the best way to achieve longer, healthier, and productive lives.

The menu suggestions beginning on page 156 are broken down into two categories. The first 7-day menu (physically inactive) suggestions are for those who will be doing little to no exercise. The second 7-day menu (physically active) suggestions are for those who are involved in a vigorous exercise program. For that reason the second menu suggestions provide for a greater intake of protein, for all the prior reasons explained.

It should be noted that almost all of the menu items listed do not require extensive cooking skills. This is because the authors believe most of the food you eat should not and does not require cooking to be healthy. From the outset it may appear quite Spartan to eat foods in the forms suggested, but research has shown the less complicated your menu the more likely you are stay with the diet, and less likely you are to add ingredients for taste that are not good for you.

It is hoped, as the menus suggest, that the majority of foods can be bought and prepared with the least amount of cooking and preparation. In addition, it is suggested you eat as much organic food as possible, and foods in their natural state, to preserve the vitamins and minerals inherent in these foods. In some cases this may cause some of your food costs to go up, but in the long run, it is just better for your health to eat unprocessed or "fast foods."

Please note that when the authors list, as an example, coffee, many people add milk or cream. However, where Blood Type A is concerned it is suggested you drink the coffee black or with soymilk. In no event do the authors suggest using any dairy product, even in small amounts. As to sweeteners, it is suggested you refer to your list of acceptable foods; however artificial sweeteners such as Nutrasweet and Aspartame are acceptable in small amounts. Although the above sweeteners have come under attack, it is an historical fact that the FDA required more than 100 studies, more than any other products, prior to approval.

When the authors suggest peanut butter they are referring only to organic peanut butter. Store bought brands contains ingredients which in most cases are contraindicated for your health. When the authors refer to using eggs for Type As, it is suggested organic eggs be used whenever possible.

When the authors provide a menu for Type A and AB, it is suggested that each morning begin with a four-ounce glass of luke-warm water with 1/2 squeezed lemon. This will help remove any overnight congestion that may have occurred, followed ten minutes later by a six-ounce glass of non-sweetened grapefruit juice. The grapefruit juice becomes alkaline in the stomach of Type As and ABs, which is beneficial prior to eating other foods. When the A and AB are in the alkaline state the metabolism of food is natural and more efficient. So although it is suggested each day for As and ABs, it will only appear on the first day's menu for each blood type.

As you will note by the outlined menus, it is recommended you eat three regular meals, an afternoon snack, and a protein shake at breakfast and before bedtime. The schedule was planned in order to insure that you do not become hungry so as to disturb your hormone balance during the day. The protein shakes are intended to ensure you receive the highest quality protein for your body. Also, the protein shake before bed places your body in an anabolic state which, if you will remember, slows insulin production and allows you to access body fat for energy while you sleep.

If all of this seems a little overwhelming for some of you, there is hope, and its just a phone call or e-mail away. For over 30 years, Joseph Christiano has helped redesign the way Americans get into shape. He has trained Hollywood celebrities, international business executives, beauty pageant swimsuit winners, and now he can do the same for you, by mail, in the privacy of your own home.

His 90-day Interactive Home Fitness/Nutrition program is like having your own personal trainer helping you achieve your goals in the privacy of your home.

As Joe says, "Don't waste your time going to the gym, and don't fall for fad diets and lose hope." Joe will design and monitor your progress every 30 days. You'll be a changed person.

If you want Joseph Christiano to design and monitor a specific diet and exercise program just for you, he can be reached at:

Personal Nutrition USA, Inc.
P.O. Box 951479
Lake Mary, FL 32795-1479

For faster service call:
Tel: 407-332-4812
Fax : 407-260-5112
1-888-41BLOOD

Or

E-mail: bloodtype2@aol.com

The $64,000 question: **What should I eat?** This is a complicated question if you don't know what foods are best for each blood type. However, the one common denominator all blood types require for a long, healthy life is protein. But the form of protein each blood type thrives on is different and has a direct bearing on life span. **We know that Whey Protein Isolate is the superstar of protein, and has the highest biological value of any protein in nature. It is also the only protein we know of that is extremely healthy for all blood types.**

The other reason protein is so important is that there is a direct correlation between the amount of protein ingested and your glycemic index. So the next question: **What is the glycemic index and why is it important to good health?**

The glycemic index is the rate at which a carbohydrate breaks down to be released as glucose into the bloodstream. A diet too high in carbohydrates induces the secretion of insulin by the pancreas, and the suppression of glucagon. However, not all carbohydrates induce the secretion of insulin at the same rate. Therefore, the type and nature of the carbohydrate has a direct bearing on the rate of insulin secretion. For instance, sugar, a simple carbohydrate, will induce the immediate release of insulin, giving the individual an immediate burst of energy, only to lead to a crash after the body uses up the source. On the other hand, grapes, a complex carbohydrate, enters the blood stream much more slowly, providing a steady stream of energy for several hours.

Of course there are foods that contain both protein and carbohydrate, such as soybeans. Most of these foods are exceptionally healthy because they contain more protein than carbohydrate, and are very low on the glycemic index, allowing the body to remain in an anabolic state while still providing a slow steady stream of energy for the body.

To help you understand the glycemic index better, Table 15 charts many typical foods and their respective index rating. Remember, the lower the number, the slower the release of insulin into the bloodstream, which is the desired result overwhelmingly.

TABLE 15

GLYCEMIC INDEX OF COMMON FOODS

Puffed rice, Rice cakes, Puffed wheat	133
Maltose	110
Cereals	100
Glucose	100
White bread/Whole wheat	100
Carrots	92
Oat bran, rolled oats	88
Honey	87
White rice, Brown rice, Corn, Bananas	82
All bran, Kidney beans	72
Raisins, Macaroni, Beets	64
Pinto beans, Sucrose	59
Peas, Potato chips, Yams	51
Orange juice, Sweet Potatos, Sponge cake	46
Oranges, Navy Beans, Grapes, 100% Rye bread	40
Apples, Chick-peas, Ice cream, Yogurt, Milk	35
Lentils, Peaches	29
Cherries, Grapefruit, Plums	25
Soybeans	15
Peanuts	12

Please see Addendum III for a comprehensive list of foods and their respective Glycemic Index rating.

This writer believes that green soybeans (Edemame) (pronounced **Ed A Ma May**) is the healthiest food on the planet. Some people cannot tolerate soy, but the overwhelming number of all blood types can, and this assertion is based upon the following:

All Blood Types

Green Soybeans

1. Low Glycemic Index- Slow, steady stream of energy

2. Naturally Anabolic- More Protein than Carbohydrate

3. Excellent Nutrition- Protein, Carbohydrate,
                         Unsaturated Fat
                         Vitamins, Minerals,
                         Phyto/Antioxidants
                         High Fiber Food

It's not a coincidence that the Japanese eat more soybeans than any culture on earth, and they live the longest. Soy is also a natural source of estrogen, a heart disease protector for both men and women. It's not a coincidence they have such low heart disease risk profiles, and live seven (7) years longer than Americans. Among the heaviest smokers in the world, their lung cancer rate is extremely low, which we attribute to green tea containing phyto-antioxidants and polyphenols, potent cancer fighters.

Type A & AB

Unsalted, Raw, or Dry Roasted Red-skinned Peanuts

1. Low Glycemic Index, Naturally Anabolic, High in Fiber, Niacin, Folic Acid, and Resvertrol.

For A and AB, these and green soybeans are as good as it gets. In addition to the above, peanuts contain niacin that lowers cholesterol, and resvertrol, a chemical found in grape juice, red wine, and grapes, that inhibits blood clots. Since A and ABs have the greatest danger of clots by virtue of their relatively thick blood, this compound could be a lifesaver.

In addition, peanuts are high in folic acid that helps prevent birth defects in unborn children, and lowers homocystein levels. This research shows lower heart disease risks.

For most A and ABs, raw or dry-roasted red-skinned peanuts and organic peanut butter are a great source of nutrition, and extremely healthy for the heart.

Peanuts have been avoided by many for being high in fat. But of the 14 grams of fat, 12 are unsaturated. Therefore, peanuts help lower your cholesterol, raise your HDL, (good cholesterol), prevent blood clots, and are anabolic, which helps you lose weight.

But let's digress for just a minute and look at the typical American diet, which usually consists of meat and potatoes, frequently hamburgers, fries, and a soda. At least 50 million people eat this fast food regimen at least once a day, if not more often. While the meal appears balanced by virtue of the meat to provide protein, potatoes and bread for carbohydrates, oil containing fat, and soda containing carbonated water and other ingredients, the meal is unhealthy for all blood types.

The hamburger, with saturated fat, is only partially OK for type O and B. It is very unhealthy for Type A and AB, both for the meat and saturated fat content. The fries and bread provides little for Os and As, as neither is properly metabolized, and will only promote weight gain. If the bread contains sesame seeds, this could cause untold trouble for Os, Bs and ABs, in the form of diverticulitis, or gall bladder problems. And the oil, which in most cases contains more saturated rather than unsaturated fat, is harmful to all blood types. This is typical of many fast food choice meals.

Although this meal has protein, carbohydrate, and fat, it has the propensity to make all blood types ill, especially in the long run. So the answer is to provide the body with the right food in proportions that will not adversely affect your cholesterol, hormone balances, or promotes weight gain that will eventually lead to other health risks.

To begin with, fat, even saturated fat, is a neutral that doesn't affect insulin or glucagon, and will be discussed in detail later. So for illustrating my point, I will start with carbohydrates and proteins and their effect on weight and hormone levels in the body.

Every time you eat a carbohydrate your body converts it to sugar. To keep your sugar balance in check the pancreas secretes insulin to keep the body in proper balance. So in simple terms, insulin lowers your blood sugar. While this is taking place, other hormonal changes are taking place; namely, insulin is placing your body in a catabolic state, or storage mode converting protein and fat to fat. At the same time the insulin is increasing the production of cholesterol, the kidneys retain excess fluid, and glucose (sugar) is utilized for energy. The end result is weight gain. If you continue to eat carbohydrates and remain in a catabolic state indefinitely, eventually most people, except perhaps children, will gain weight, and subject themselves to diabetes, heart disease, high blood pressure, and a host of other medical problems.

Every time you eat protein the body produces glucagon and the body enters an anabolic state, or the opposite of eating carbohydrates begins. Namely, glucagon raises low blood sugar, the body shifts to a burning mode, whereby protein and fat are converted to glucose; fats are converted to ketones that are utilized for energy. Fat is released from fat cells to be used by the body for energy, and kidneys release excess water. The result is weight loss.

But in our example above and in the real world, we eat protein, fats, and carbohydrate at the same time. So the key to good health, weight loss, and the prevention of all the above-mentioned conditions is to keep the body in an anabolic state as much as possible. To do this you must eat more protein than carbohydrate as frequently as possible.

Sounds easy enough, but since the above meal is not digestible in whole or part by any blood type, and is carbohydrate heavy, the result is weight gain, and subjection to heart disease, etc. This is one reason fast foods make almost everybody fat, and increase the risks of a host of illnesses. The other reason is that improper metabolism of part or all of the food by one blood type or another slows down the body processes and further adds to weight gain.

So in reality, to achieve your best and healthiest weight you must follow the rules!

Rule 1: Eat more protein than carbohydrate as frequently as possible. This will keep your body in an anabolic state and your gylcemic index as low as possible.

Rule 2: The protein and carbohydrate you eat should be compatible with your blood type.

Rule 3: Minimize consumption of saturated fat. Consume Polyunsaturated or monounsaturated fat that is compatible with your blood type.

These are the rules, and if you follow them within the guidelines of the food groups outlined you will achieve your goals. Remember that a body in an anabolic state will not gain weight, and will continue to lose weight until the individual reaches his target weight, at which time the balance of protein to carbohydrate should be about equal.

Additionally, when you eat foods compatible with your blood type and blood enzymes, the body digests these foods naturally, and you assimilate the nutrients from these foods. After all, the goal of food is to provide the proper vitamins, minerals, micronutrients, macronutrients, including amino acids, that the body needs to function at its best.

The following food lists are intended to provide the reader the benefit of prior research that indicates which foods tend to be best suited for each blood group. However, because all individuals vary to some degree in body chemistry, your reaction to every food may vary. Only trial and error will tell which foods are best for you.

These food lists do not account for the consumption of protein, fat, and carbohydrate as they relate to the body's secretion of glucagon and insulin. For that reason the menus provided will help you with the balance to insure an anabolic state. **The first 7-day menu suggestions are for individuals who do not exercise. The second 7-day menu provides a much higher amount of protein and is intended for individuals who engage in moderate to vigorous exercise.**

As you review the food lists keep in mind that the beneficial foods tend to metabolize faster and easier, because of blood enzymes. Conversely, avoid foods that do not digest or metabolize well, and thus disrupt normal metabolism. It is for this reason we suggest that when you start this regimen you eat as many foods from the beneficial food groups as possible, slowly adding neutral foods as you gravitate to your target weight.

GROCERY LISTS & DIET PLAN FOR MAXIMUM LIFE

Also, since you will probably be eating more protein than you have on a regular basis, remember to drink plenty of water throughout the day. This is essential because your kidneys require more water to metabolize protein, and because water is the universal solvent and aids digestion of all foods in general. So when in doubt, drink more water. **As a rule of thumb** divide your body weight by 1/2, then convert the pounds to ounces of water. Now you have the amount you should be drinking each day. **Example: 150 lbs. x 1/2 = 75** ounces of water per day. Obviously, if you engage in intense physical exercise your requirements will be higher. When you consider that the human body is comprised of 75% water, the brain 90%, and all enzymes, digestion, and other bodily functions which require water, it just makes sense to give your body what it needs most.

While the following lists of foods for each blood group are not written in stone, this research provides the foundation for a blueprint of foods best suited for each blood type.

When you review your particular list, if some of your favorite foods appear on your avoid list, we're sorry. It's just a matter of chemistry, and the rules are the rules. This is not to say there are not exceptions to the rule, as in every population this is true. However, we suggest you follow the rules as closely as possible, and monitor your results to maximize your benefits.

Although many test subjects followed the recommended diet, and still do, we have published one subject who is 52 and came from a family in which his father and sister died of fatal heart attacks at early ages, and one parent lives with heart disease. His blood tests are very gratifying, but you decide for yourself.

TABLE 16

BLOOD PRESSURE/CHOLESTEROL COMPARISON

		Normal
Blood Pressure before diet and exercise	140/95	120/80
Blood Pressure after diet and exercise	115/75	
Cholesterol 5 years prior	291	120-200
Cholesterol before diet and exercise	243	
Cholesterol after diet and exercise	140	
HDL 5 years prior	35	35-95
HDL before	45	
HDL after	62	
HDL/Cholesterol Ratio 5 years ago (high risk)	8.3	3.5-11
HDL/Cholesterol Ratio 2 years ago	4.74	
HDL/Cholesterol Ratio after (lowest 1% risk)	2.25*	
LDL before (bad cholesterol)	232	50-130
LDL after (bad cholesterol)	79	
Triglicerides 5 years prior (fat in the blood)	232	40-200
Triglicerides after diet and exercise	41	

*The lower the ratio, the lower the heart disease risk.

Blood Type A

Grocery list of very beneficial foods

(A) After foods designates which are anabolic

**Anabolic- Higher in Protein than Carbohydrate
(All meats and seafood are naturally anabolic)**

Meats/Seafood (There are no beneficial meats)
Seafood- Carp, Cod, Grouper, Mackerel, Monkfish, Pickerel, Rainbow trout, Snapper, Ocean Salmon, Sardine, Sea trout, Silver perch, Snail, Whitefish, Yellow perch **(A)**

Eggs/Dairy
Soy cheese **(A)**, Soy milk, **Whey Protein Isolate (A)**

Oils/Fats/Nuts/Seeds
Linseed/Flaxseed oil, Olive oil, Macadamia nuts, Organic peanut butter **(A)**, Unsalted-red-skinned peanuts **(A)**, Pumpkin seeds

Beans and Legumes
Aduke, Azuki, Black, Green, Pinto, Soy beans (Black, Brown, (Green-Edemame) **(A)**, Lentils (domestic, green, and red), Black-eyed peas

Cereals/Bread/Grains/Pasta
Amaranth, Buckwheat, Kasha, Essene bread, Ezekiel bread, Soy flour, Sprouted wheat, Puffed rice, Rice cakes, Flour (oat, rice, rye), Soba noodles, Spelt noodles, Artichoke pasta

Vegetables/Fruits/Juices
Artichokes, Beet leaves, Broccoli, Broccoli sprouts, Carrots, Chicory, Collard greens, Okra, Onions (red, Spanish, yellow), Parsley, Parsnips, Pumpkin, Dandelion, Escarole, Garlic, Horseradish, Kohlrabi, Leek, Romaine lettuce, Spinach, Alfalfa sprouts, Swiss chard, Tempeh **(A)**, Tofu **(A)**, Turnips, **Fruits-** Apricot, Blackberries, Blueberries, Boysenberries, Cherries, Cranberries, Figs (dried and fresh), Grapefruit, Kiwi, Lemons, Pineapple, Plums (dark, green, red), Prunes, Raisins, **Juices-** Apricot, Black Cherry, Carrot, Celery, Grapefruit, Pineapple, Prune, Water & lemon

Spices/Condiments

Mustard, Barley malt, Blackstrap molasses, Garlic, Ginger, Miso, Soy sauce, Tamari

Beverages/Herbal Teas

Bottled Water, Coffee (regular and decaf), Red wine, <u>Tea-</u> Green tea, Alfalfa, Aloe, Burdock, Chamomile, Echinacea, Fenugreek, Ginger, Ginseng, Hawthorn, Milk thistle, Rose hips, Saint Johns Wort, Slippery Elm, Valerian

<u>NOTE: Whey Protein Isolate is extremely beneficial for all blood types. Medical research has shown Whey Protein Isolate boosts the immune systems of individuals whose immune systems are impaired or compromised.</u>

Blood Type A

Grocery list of neutral foods

(A) Meats/Seafood · all anabolic

Chicken, Cornish hens, Turkey, **Seafood-** Abalone, Mahi-mahi, Ocean perch, Pike, Porgy, Sailfish, Sea bass, Shark, Smelt, Sturgeon, Swordfish, Tuna, Weakfish, White perch, Yellowtail

Eggs/Dairy

Eggs **(A)** Farmer cheese **(A)**, Feta cheese **(A)**, Goat's cheese **(A)**, Mozzarella **(A)**, Ricotta **(A)**, String cheese **(A)**, Goat milk, Kefir, Yogurt

Oils/Fats/Nuts/Seeds

Canola oil, Cod liver oil, Almond butter **(A)**, Chestnuts, Filbert **(A)**, Hickory **(A)**, Litchi, Pine, Poppy seeds, Sesame seeds, Sunflower butter, Sunflower seeds, Tahini, Walnuts **(A)**

Beans and Legumes

Broad, Cannellini, Fava, Jicama, Snap, String, White, Peas (green, pod, snow).

Cereals/Bread/Grains/Pasta

Barley, Cornflakes, Cornmeal, Corn muffins, Kamut, Millet, Oat bran, Oatmeal, Oat bran muffins, Rice bran, Cream of Rice, Puffed rice, Brown rice, Rice (basmati, brown, white, wild), Spelt, Spelt noodles, Spelt pasta, Wheat bagels, Gluten free bread, Hi-protein No Wheat bread, Ideal flat bread, 100% Rye bread, Rye Crisp, Rye Vita, Wasa, Fin Crisp, Couscous, Flour (barley, bulgur wheat, durum wheat, gluten, graham, spelt, sprouted wheat), Quinoa

Vegetables

Arugula, Asparagus, Florida Avocado, Bamboo shoots, Beets, Bok choy, Caraway, Cauliflower, Celery, Chervil, Coriander, White corn, Yellow corn, Mushroom tree oyster, Mustard greens, Green olives, Green onions, Radicchio, Cucumber, Daikon Radish, Endive, Fennel, Ferns, Kale, Lettuce (bibb, iceberg, mesclun), Mushrooms (abalone, enoki, portobello), Radishes, Rappini, Rutabaga, Scallion, Seaweed, Shallots, Sprouts (brussel, mung, radish), All types of Squash, Water Chestnut, Watercress, Zucchini

Fruits/Juices

Apples, Black currants, Red currants, Dates, Elderberries, Gooseberries, Grapes (black, concord, green, red), Guava, Kumquat, Limes, Loganberries, Melon (canang, casaba, Christmas, crenshaw, musk, Spanish), Watermelon, Nectarines, Peaches, Pears, Persimmons, Pomegranates, Prickly Pears, Raspberries, Starfruit, Strawberries, **Juices-** Apple cider, Apple juice, Cabbage juice, Cranberry juice, Cucumber juice, Grape juice, Vegetable juice

Spices/Condiments

Agar, Allspice, Almond extract, Anise, Arrowroot, Basil, Bay leaf, Bergamot, Brown rice syrup, Cardamom, Carob, Chervil, Chives, Chocolate, Cinnamon, Clove, Coriander, Corn syrup, Cornstarch, Cream of tartar, Cumin, Curry, Dill, Dulse, Honey, Horseradish, Kelp, Maple syrup, Mint, Mustard dry, Nutmeg, Oregano, Paprika, Parsley, Peppermint, Pimiento, Rice syrup, Rosemary, Saffron, Sage, Salt, Savory, Spearmint, Brown sugar, White sugar, Tamarind, Tapioca, Tarragon, Thyme, Turmeric, Vanilla, Jam/Jelly for approved fruits, Pickles (dill, kosher, sour, sweet), Relish

Beverages/Herbal Teas

Seltzer Water, Soda Water, White wine, **Tea-** Chickweed, Colts foot, Dandelion, Dong Quai, Elder, Gent Ian, Goldenseal, Hops, Horehound, Licorice, Linden, Mulberry, Mullein, Parsley, Peppermint, Raspberry Leaf, Sage, Sarsaparilla, Senna, Shepherd's purse, Skullcap, Spearmint, Strawberry Leaf, Thyme, Vervain, White birch, White oak bark, Yarrow

Blood Type A

List of avoid foods

Note: Most Blood Type A people should be vegetarian: there are no beneficial meats. All meat should be avoided in favor of poultry, which is neutral.
No anabolic foods are designated on avoid list

Meats/Seafood
Beef, Buffalo, Duck, Goose, Heart, Lamb, Liver, Mutton, Partridge, Pheasant, All Pork, Rabbit, Veal, Venison, Quail, **Seafood-** Anchovy, Barracuda, Beluga, Bluefish, Bluegill bass, Catfish, Caviar, Clam, Conch, Crab, Crayfish, Eel, Flounder, Frog, Gray Sole, Haddock, Hake, Halibut, Herring (fresh or pickled), Lobster, Lox, Mussels, Octopus, Oysters, Scallop, Shad, Shrimp, Sole, Squid, Striped bass, Tilefish, Turtle

Eggs/Dairy
American cheese, Blue cheese, Brie, Butter, Buttermilk, Camembert, Casein, Cheddar, Colby, Cottage, Cream Cheese, Edam, Emmenthal, Gouda, Gruyere, Ice cream, Jarlsberg, Monterey Jack, Muenster, Neufchatel, Parmesan, Provolone, Sherbet, Skim or 2% milk, Sour cream (non-fat), Swiss, Whole milk

Oils/Fats/Nuts/Seeds
Corn oil, Cottonseed oil, Peanut oil, Safflower oil, Sesame oil, Brazil nuts, Cashews, Pistachios

Beans and Legumes
Copper, Garbanzo, Kidney, Lima, Navy, Red, Tamarind

Cereals/Bread/Grains/Pasta
Cream of wheat, Familia, Farina, Granola, Grape nuts, Wheat germs, Seven grain, Shredded wheat, Wheat bran, Durum wheat, English muffins, High-protein bread, Wheat matzos, Pumpernickel, Wheat bran muffins, Whole wheat bread, Whole wheat and white flour, Semolina pasta, Spinach pasta

Vegetables/Fruits/Juices

Chinese, Red and White Cabbage, Eggplant, Domestic and Shitake mushrooms, Black, Greek and Spanish Olives, Green, Red, Yellow and Jalapeño Peppers, Sweet, Red, and White Potatoes, Yams, Tomatoes, **Fruits** Bananas, Coconuts, Mangoes, Cantaloupe and Honeydew Melon, Oranges, Papayas, Plantains, Rhubarb, Tangerines, **Juices** Orange, Papaya, Tomato

Spices/Condiments

Caper; Gelatin; Black, Cayenne, Peppercorn, Red and White Pepper; Apple cider, Balsamic, Red or white Vinegar; Wintergreen, Ketchup; Mayonnaise; Tabasco sauce, Worcestershire sauce

Beverages

Beer, Liquor, Sodas, Black tea (regular or decaf)

Blood Type B

Grocery list of very beneficial foods

(A) After foods designates which are anabolic

Anabolic- Higher in Protein than Carbohydrate

Meats/Seafood- all anabolic

Lamb, Rabbit, Venison, **Seafood-** Caviar, Cod, Grouper, Haddock, Hake, Halibut, Mackerel, Mahi-mahi, Monkfish, Ocean perch, Pickerel, Pike, Porgy, Sardine, Sea trout, Shad, Sole, Sturgeon

Eggs/Dairy

Cottage cheese **(A)**, Farmer cheese **(A)**, Feta cheese **(A)**, Goat cheese **(A)**, Mozzarella cheese **(A)**, Ricotta cheese **(A)**, Goat milk, Kefir, Skim or 2% milk, **Whey Protein Isolate (A)**, Yogurt

Oils/Fats/Nuts/Seeds

Olive oil, Macadamia nuts

Beans and Legumes

Kidney, Lima, Navy, Soy beans (Black, Brown, Green-Edemame) **(A)**

Cereals/Bread/Grains/Pasta

Oat bran, Oatmeal, Oat flour, Rice bran, Puffed rice, Rice cakes, Rice flour, Rice pasta, Millet, Puffed millet, Spelt, Spelt pasta, Brown rice bread, Essence bread, Ezekiel bread, Wasa bread, Fin Crisp

Vegetables/Fruits/Juices

Florida Avocado, Beets, Beet leaves, Broccoli, Cabbage (Chinese, red, white), Carrots, Cauliflower, Collard greens, Eggplant, Kale, Lima beans, Shitake Mushroom, Mustard greens, Parsley, Parsnips, Peppers (green, jalapeño, red, yellow), Sweet potatoes, Brussel sprouts, Yams **Fruits-** Cranberries, Grapes (black, concord, green, red), Kiwi, Papaya, Pineapple, Plums (dark, green, red) **Juices-** Cabbage, Cranberry, Grape, Papaya, Pineapple

Spices/Condiments
Cayenne pepper, Curry, Ginger, Horseradish, Parsley

Beverages/Herbal teas
Bottled Water, Red wine, **Tea-** Green tea, Ginger, Ginseng, Licorice, Parsley, Peppermint, Raspberry leaf, Rose hips, Sage

NOTE: Whey Protein Isolate is extremely beneficial for all blood types. Medical research has shown Whey Protein Isolate boosts the immune systems of individuals whose immune systems are impaired or compromised.

Blood Type B

Grocery list of neutral foods

Meats/Seafood- all anabolic

Beef, Ground beef, Buffalo, Liver, Pheasant, Turkey, Veal, **Seafood-** Abalone, Bluefish, Carp, Catfish, Smelt, Herring, Rainbow trout, Red snapper, Sailfish, Ocean Salmon, Scallop, Shark, Silver perch, Snapper, Squid, Swordfish, Tilefish, Tuna, Whitefish, White perch, Yellow perch

Eggs/Dairy

Eggs **(A)** Butter, Buttermilk, Brie **(A)** Camembert **(A)** Casein **(A)**, Cheddar **(A)**, Colby **(A)**, Cream cheese **(A)**, Edam **(A)**, Emmenthal **(A)**, Gouda **(A)**, Gruyere **(A)**, Jarlsberg **(A)**, Monterey Jack **(A)**, Muenster **(A)**, Neufchatel **(A)**, Parmesan **(A)**, Provolone **(A)**, Soy cheese **(A)**, Swiss **(A)**, Sherbet, Soy milk, Regular Whey **(A)**, Whole milk

Oils/Fats/Nuts/Seeds

Cod liver oil, Linseed (flaxseed oil), Almond butter **(A)**, Almonds **(A)**, Brazil nuts **(A)**, Chestnuts, Hickory **(A)**, Litchi, Pecans

Beans and Legumes

Broad, Cannellini, Copper, Fava, Green, Jicama, Northern, Red, Snap, String, Tamarind, White, Peas (green, pod, snow)

Cereals/Bread/Grains/Pasta

Cream of rice, Familia, Farina, Granola, Grape nuts, Gluten free bread, Hi-protein no wheat bread, Ideal flat, Pumpernickel, Soy flour, Spelt, Oat bran muffins, Graham flour, White flour, Pasta semolina, Pasta spinach, Quinoa, Rice (basmati, brown, white)

Vegetables

Arugula, Asparagus, Bok choy, Celery, Chervil, Chicory, Cucumber, Daikon radish, Dandelion, Dill, Endive, Escarole, Fennel, Fiddlehead Ferns, Garlic, Ginger, Horseradish, Kohlrabi, Leek, Lettuce (bibb, boston, iceberg, mesclun, romaine), Mushrooms (abalone, domestic, enoki, portobello, tree oyster), Okra, Onions (green, red, spanish, yellow), Potatoes (red and white), Radicchio, Rappini, Rutabaga, Scallion, Seaweed, Shallots, Spinach, Alfalfa sprouts, Squash (all types), Swiss chard, Turnips, Water chestnut, Watercress, Zucchini

Fruits/Juices

Apples, Apricots, Bananas, Blackberries, Blueberries, Boysenberries, Cherries, Currants (red and black), Dates, Elderberries, Figs (fresh and dried), Gooseberries, Grapefruit, Guava, Kumquat, Lemons, Limes, Loganberries, Mangoes, Melon- all varieties, Watermelon, Nectarines, Oranges, Peaches, Prunes, Raisins, Raspberries, Strawberries, Tangerines, **Juices** Apple cider, Apple, Apricot, Black Cherry, Carrot, Celery, Cucumber, Grapefruit, Orange, Prune, Water & lemon

Spices/Condiments

Apple butter, Jelly/Jam of approved fruits, Mayonnaise, Mustard, Pickles (dill, kosher, sour, sweet), Relish, Salad dressing, Worcestershire sauce, Agar, Allspice, Anise, Arrowroot, Basil, Bay leaf, Bergamot, Brown rice syrup, Caraway, Cardamom, Carob, Chervil, Chives, Chocolate, Clove, Coriander, Corn syrup, Cream of tartar, Cumin, Curry, Dill, Dulse, Honey, Horseradish, Kelp, Maple syrup, Mint, Molasses, Mustard dry, Nutmeg, Oregano, Paprika, Parsley, Peppermint, Pimiento, Rice syrup, Rosemary, Saffron, Sage, Salt, Savory, Spearmint, White and Brown sugar, Tabasco sauce, Tamarind, Tarragon, Thyme, Turmeric, Vanilla, Vinegar (apple cider, balsamic, red wine, white), Wintergreen

Beverages/Herbal teas

Seltzer Water, Soda Water, Beer, Regular and decaf coffee, Regular and decaf **Tea-** Black tea, Red and White wine, Alfalfa, Burdock, Catnip, Cayenne, Chamomile, Chickweed, Dandelion, Dong Quai, Echinacea, Elder, Goldenseal, Green tea, Hawthorn, Horehound, Mulberry, Saint Johns Wort, Sarsaparilla, Slippery Elm, Spearmint, Strawberry leaf, Thyme, Valerian, Vervain, White birch, White oak bark, Yarrow, Yellow dock

Blood Type B

List of avoid foods

No anabolic foods are designated on avoid list

Meats/Seafood

Chicken, Cornish hens, Duck, Goose, Heart, Partridge, All Pork, Quail, **Seafood-** Anchovy, Barracuda, Beluga, Bluegill bass, Clam, Conch, Crab, Crayfish, Eel, Frog, Lobster, Lox, Mussels, Octopus, Oysters, Farm Raised Salmon, Sea Bass, Shrimp, Snail, Striped bass, Turtle, Yellowtail

Eggs/Dairy

American cheese, Blue cheese, Ice cream, String cheese

Oils/Fats/Nuts/Seeds

Canola oil, Corn oil, Cottonseed oil, Peanut oil, Safflower oil, Sesame oil, Sunflower oil, Cashews, Filberts, Pignola, Pistachio, Peanuts, Peanut butter, Poppy seeds, Pumpkin seeds, Sesame butter (tahini) and seeds, Sunflower seeds

Beans and Legumes

Aduke; Azuki; Black; Garbanzo; Pinto; Domestic, Green and Red Lentils; Black-eyed Peas

Cereals/Bread/Grains/Pasta

Amaranth, Barley, Buckwheat, Cornflakes, Cornmeal, Cream of wheat, Gluten Flour, Kamut, Kasha, Rye, Seven-grain, Shredded wheat, Soba Noodles, Wheat bran, Wheat germ, Wheat bagels, Corn muffins, Durum wheat, Multi-grain bread, 100% rye bread, Rye crisp, Rye Vita, Wheat bran muffins, Whole wheat flour, Buckwheat, Couscous, Artichoke Pasta, Wild Rice

Vegetables/Fruits

Domestic and Jerusalem Artichoke, CA Avocado, White and Yellow Corn, Black, Green, Greek and Spanish Olives, Pumpkin, Radishes, Mung Sprouts, Tempeh, Tofu, Tomato, **Fruits-** Coconuts, Persimmons, Pomegranate, Prickly Pear, Rhubarb, Starfruit

Spices/Condiments

Allspice, Almond extract, Barley malt, Capers, Cinnamon, Cornstarch, Corn syrup, Plain Gelatin, Ketchup, Black ground and White Pepper, Tapioca

Beverages

Distilled liquor, Sodas

Blood Type AB

Grocery list of very beneficial foods

(A) After foods designates which are anabolic

**Anabolic - Higher in Protein than Carbohydrate
(All meats and seafood are naturally anabolic)**

Meats/Seafood - All anabolic
Rabbit, Turkey, **Seafood-** Cod, Grouper, Hake, Mackerel, Mahi-mahi, Monkfish, Ocean perch, Pickerel, Pike, Porgy, Rainbow trout, Ocean Salmon, Snapper, Sailfish, Sardine, Sea trout, Shad, Snail, Sturgeon, Tuna

Eggs/Dairy
Non-fat Cottage cheese **(A)** Farmer cheese **(A)**, Feta cheese **(A)**, Goat cheese **(A)**, Mozzarella **(A)**, Ricotta cheese **(A)**, Non-fat Sour cream, **Whey Protein Isolate (A)***, Yogurt

Oils/Fats/Nuts/Seeds
Olive oil, Chestnuts, Macadamia nuts, Organic peanut butter **(A)**, Unsalted red-skinned peanuts **(A)**, Walnuts **(A)**

Beans and Legumes
Green lentils, Navy, Pinto, Red, Soy (Black, Brown, Green-Edemame) **(A)**

Cereals/Bread/Grains/Pasta
Essene bread, Ezekiel bread, Oat bran, Oatmeal, Oat flour, Rice bran, Puffed rice, Rice cakes, Brown rice bread, Rice pasta, Millet, Puffed millet, 100% Rye bread, 100% Rye flour, Rye crisp, Vita Rye, Spelt, Spelt pasta, Soy flour

Vegetables/Fruits/Juices

Florida Avocado, Beet leaves, Beets, Broccoli, Broccoli sprouts, Cauliflower, Celery, Collard greens, Cucumber, Dandelion, Eggplant, Garlic, Mustard greens, Parsley, Parsnips, Sweet potatoes, Alfalfa sprouts, Tempeh **(A)**, Tofu **(A)**, Yams **Fruits** Cherries, Cranberries, Figs (dried and fresh), Gooseberries, Grapefruit, Grapes (black, concord, green, red), Kiwi, Lemons, Loganberries, Pineapple, Plums (dark, green, red) **Juices** Black Cherry, Cabbage, Carrot, Celery, Cranberry, Grape, Papaya

Spices/Condiments

Curry, Garlic, Horseradish, Miso, Parsley

Beverages/Herbal Teas

Bottled Water, Coffee (regular and decaf), Red wine, **Tea-** Green tea, Alfalfa, Burdock, Chamomile, Echinacea, Ginger, Ginseng, Hawthorn, Licorice, Milk thistle, Rose hips, Strawberry leaf

<u>NOTE: Whey Protein Isolate is extremely beneficial for all blood types. Medical research has shown Whey Protein Isolate boosts the immune systems of individuals whose immune systems are impaired or compromised.</u>

Blood Type AB

Grocery list of neutral foods

Meats/Seafood - all anabolic

Lamb, Liver, Pheasant, Seafood- Abalone, Bluefish, Carp, Catfish, Caviar, Fresh herring, Mussels, Scallop, Shark, Silver perch, Smelt, Sole, Squid, Swordfish, Tilefish, Weakfish, White perch, Whitefish, Yellow perch

Eggs/Dairy

Eggs **(A)** Casein cheese **(A)**, Cheddar cheese **(A)**, Colby cheese **(A)**, Cream cheese **(A)**, Edam **(A)**, Emmenthal **(A)**, Gouda **(A)**, Gruyere **(A)**, Jarlsberg **(A)**, Monterey Jack **(A)**, Muenster **(A)**, Neufchatel **(A)**, Soy **(A)**, String **(A)**, Swiss **(A)**, Goat Milk, Kefir, Skim or 2% milk, Soy milk, Regular Whey **(A)**

Oils/Fats/Nuts/Seeds

Canola oil, Cod liver oil, Linseed (flaxseed) oil, Peanut oil, Almond butter **(A)**, Almonds **(A)**, Brazil nuts **(A)**, Cashews, Hickory **(A)**, Litchi, Pine, Pistachios

Beans and Legumes

Broad, Cannelloni, Copper, Green, Jicama, Northern, Snap, String, Tamarind, White, Lentils (domestic, red), Peas (green, pod, snow)

Cereals/Bread/Grains/Pasta

Amaranth, Barley, Cream of Rice, Cream of Wheat, Familia, Farina, Granola, Grape nuts, Seven Grain, Shredded wheat, Soy flakes, Soy granules, Wheat bran, Wheat germ, Wheat bagels, Gluten free bread, Hi-protein bread, Ideal flat bread, Multi-grain bread, Pumpernickel, Spelt, Whole wheat, Durum wheat, English muffins, Oat bran muffins, Wheat bran muffins, Wheat matzos, Couscous, Flour (barley, bulgur wheat, durum wheat, gluten, graham, spelt, white, whole wheat), Semolina pasta, Spinach pasta, Quinoa

Vegetables/Fruits/Juices

Arugula, Asparagus, Bamboo shoots, Bok choy, Cabbage (chinese, red, white), Caraway, Carrots, Chervil, Chicory, Coriander, Daikon, Endive, Escarole, Fennel, Fiddlehead Ferns, Ginger, Horseradish, Kohlrabi, Leek, Lettuce (bibb, Boston, iceberg, mesclun, romaine), Mushrooms (domestic, enoki, portobello, tree oyster), Okra, Olives (greek, green, spanish), Onions (green, red, spanish, yellow), Red potatoes, White potatoes, Pumpkin, Radicchio, Rappini, Rutabaga, Scallion, Seaweed, Shallots, Spinach, Brussel sprouts, Squash-all types, Swiss chard, Tomato, Turnips, Water Chestnut, Watercress, Zucchini **Fruits** Apples, Apricots, Blackberries, Blueberries, Boysenberries, Black currants, Red currants, Dates, Elderberries, Kumquat, Limes, Melon- all types, Watermelon, Nectarines, Papaya, Peaches, Pears, Plantains, Prunes, Raisins, Raspberries, Strawberries, Tangerines **Juices** Apple cider, Apple juice, Apricot juice, Cucumber juice, Grapefruit juice, Pineapple juice, Prune juice, Vegetable juice, Water & lemon

Spices/Condiments

Agar, Arrowroot, Basil, Bay leaf, Bergamot, Brown rice syrup, Cardamom, Carob, Chervil, Chives, Chocolate, Cinnamon, Clove, Coriander, Cream of tartar, Cumin, Dill, Dulse, Honey, Kelp, Maple syrup, Marjoram, Mint, Molasses, Mustard dry, Nutmeg, Paprika, Peppermint, Pimiento, Rice syrup, Rosemary, Saffron, Sage, Salt, Savory, Soy sauce, Spearmint, Brown sugar, White sugar, Tamari, Tamarind, Tarragon, Thyme, Turmeric, Vanilla, Wintergreen

Beverages/Herbal Teas

Beer, Seltzer water, Club soda, White wine, **Tea** Catnip, Cayenne, Chickweed, Dandelion, Dong Quai, Elder, Goldenseal, Horehound, Mulberry, Parsley, Peppermint, Raspberry Leaf, Sage, Saint Johns Wort, Sarsaparilla, Slippery Elm, Spearmint, Thyme, Valerian, Vervain, White birch, White oak bark, Yarrow, Yellow dock

Blood Type AB

List of avoid foods

No anabolic foods designated on avoid list

Meats/Seafood

Beef, Buffalo, Chicken, Cornish hens, Duck, Goose, Heart, Partridge, All Pork, Veal, Venison, Quail, **Seafood-** Anchovy, Barracuda, Beluga, Bluegill bass, Clam, Conch, Crab, Crayfish, Eel, Flounder, Frog, Gray sole, Haddock, Halibut, Pickled Herring, Lobster, Lox, Octopus, Oysters, Farm Raised Salmon, Sea Bass, Shrimp, Striped bass, Turtle, Yellowtail

Eggs/Dairy

American cheese, Blue cheese, Brie, Butter, Buttermilk, Camembert, Ice cream, Parmesan, Provolone, Sherbet, Whole Milk

Oils/Fats/Nuts/Seeds

Corn oil, Cottonseed oil, Safflower oil, Sesame oil, Sunflower oil, Filberts, Poppy seeds, Pumpkin seeds, Sesame seeds & butter (tahini), Sunflower seeds

Beans and Legumes

Aduke, Azuki, Black, Fava, Garbanzo, Kidney, Lima, Black-eyed Peas

Cereals/Bread/Grains/Pasta

Buckwheat, Corn, Kamut, Kasha, Corn muffins, Artichoke Pasta, Soba Noodles

Vegetables/Fruits

Domestic and Jerusalem Artichoke, CA Avocado, White and Yellow Corn, Abalone and Shitake Mushrooms, Black Olives, Green, Red, Yellow and Jalapeño Peppers, Radishes, Radish Sprouts, Mung Sprouts, **Fruits-** Bananas, Coconuts, Guava, Mangoes, Oranges, Persimmons, Pomegranate, Prickly Pear, Rhubarb, Starfruit

Spices/Condiments

Allspice, Almond extract, Anise, Barley malt, Capers, Cornstarch, Corn syrup, Black, Cayenne, Pepper (black, cayenne, red flakes, peppercorn), Tapioca, Vinegar (balsamic, red or white), Ketchup, Pickles (kosher, sweet, sour), Relish, Worcestershire sauce

Beverages

Distilled liquor, Sodas, Black tea

Blood Type O

Grocery list of very beneficial foods

(A) After foods designates which are anabolic

Anabolic - Higher in Protein than Carbohydrate

Meats/Seafood (A) (All are anabolic)

Beef, Ground beef, Buffalo, Heart, Lamb, Liver, Mutton, Veal, Venison, **Seafood-** Bluefish, Cod, Hake, Halibut, Fresh Herring, Mackerel, Pike, Rainbow trout, Red snapper, Salmon, Sardines, Shad, Snapper, Sole, Striped bass, Sturgeon, Swordfish, Tilefish, White perch, Whitefish, Yellow perch, Yellowtail **(A)**

Eggs/Dairy

Mozzarella cheese- non-fat, Sour cream- non-fat, **Whey Protein Isolate** **(A)***

Oils/Fats/Nuts/Seeds

Linseed (flaxseed) oil, Olive oil, Macadamia nuts, Pumpkin seeds, Walnuts **(A)**

Beans and Legumes

Aduke, Azuki, Black-eyed peas, Pinto beans

Cereals/Bread/Grains/Pasta

Essene bread, Ezekiel bread

Vegetables/Fruits/Juices

Domestic and Jerusalem Artichoke, Florida Avocado, Beet leaves, Broccoli, Broccoli sprouts, Chicory, Collard greens, Dandelion, Escarole, Garlic, Horseradish, Kale, Kohlrabi, Leek, Romaine lettuce, Okra, Onions (red, Spanish, yellow), Parsley, Parsnips, Red peppers, Sweet potatoes, Pumpkin, Seaweed, Spinach, Swiss chard, Turnips, **Fruits-** Dried and fresh Figs, Kiwi, Plums (dark, green, red), Prunes **Juices-** Black Cherry, Pineapple, Prune

Spices/Condiments
Carob, Curry, Dulse, Kelp, Parsley, Cayenne pepper, Tabasco, Turmeric

Beverages/Herbal Teas
Bottled Water, Seltzer water, Soda water, Red wine, **Tea**- Cayenne, Chickweed, Dandelion, Fenugreek, Ginger, Green tea, Hops, Linden, Milk thistle, Mulberry, Parsley, Peppermint, Rose hips, Sarsaparilla, Slippery Elm

NOTE: Whey Protein Isolate is extremely beneficial for all blood types. Medical research has shown Whey Protein Isolate boosts the immune systems of individuals whose immune systems are impaired or compromised.

Blood Type O

Grocery list of neutral foods

Meats/Seafood - all anabolic

Chicken, Cornish hens, Duck, Partridge, Pheasant, Quail, Rabbit, Turkey, **Seafood-** Abalone, Anchovy, Beluga, Bluegill bass, Carp, Clam, Crab, Crayfish, Frog, Gray sole, Grouper, Haddock, Lobster, Mahi-mahi, Monkfish, Mussels, Ocean perch, Oysters, Pickerel, Porgy, Sailfish, Scallop, Sea bass, Sea trout, Shark, Shrimp, Silver perch, Smelt, Snail, Squid, Tuna, Turtle **(A)**

Eggs/Dairy

Eggs **(A)**, Butter, Farmer cheese **(A)**, Feta cheese **(A)**, Goat cheese **(A)**, Mozzarella **(A)**, Soy cheese **(A)**, Soy milk

Oils/Fats/Nuts/Seeds

Canola oil, Cod liver oil, Sesame oil, Almond butter **(A)**, Chestnuts, Filberts **(A)**, Hickory **(A)**, Pecans, Pine, Sesame seeds, Sunflower butter, Sunflower seeds, Tahini

Beans and Legumes

Black, Broad, Cannelloni, Fava, Garbanzo, Green, Jicama, Lima, Northern, Red, Soy (Black, Brown, Green- Edemame) **(A)**, Snap, String, White, Peas (green, snow, pod)

Cereals/Bread/Grains/Pasta

Amaranth, Barley, Buckwheat, Cream of rice, Rice cakes, Kamut, Kasha, Millet, Rice bran, Puffed rice, Rice (basmati, brown, white, wild), Brown rice bread, Spelt, Spelt bread, Gluten free bread, Ideal flat bread, 100% Rye bread, Soy flour bread, Wasa, Fin Crisp, Millet,, Rye crisp, Rye vita, Flour (barley, buckwheat, rice, rye, spelt), Artichoke pasta, Quinoa

Vegetables

Arugula, Asparagus, Bamboo shoots, Beets, Bok choy, Caraway, Carrots, Celery, Chervil, Coriander, Cucumber, Daikon, Dill, Endive, Fennel, Fiddlehead Ferns, Ginger, Lettuce (bibb, Boston, iceberg, mesclun), Mushrooms (enoki, portobello, tree oyster), Green olives, Green onions, Peppers (green, jalapeño, yellow), Radicchio, Radishes, Rappini, Rutabaga, Scallion, Shallots, Sprouts (mung and radish), All types of Squash, Tempeh **(A)**, Tofu **(A)**, Tomato, Water chestnut, Watercress, Yams, Zucchini

Fruits/Juices

Apples, Apricots, Bananas, Blueberries, Boysenberries, Cherries, Cranberries, Black and Red Currants, Dates, Elderberries, Gooseberries, Grapefruit, Grapes (black, concord, green, red), Guava, Kumquat, Lemons, Limes, Loganberries, Mangoes, Melons (casaba, Christmas, crenshaw, musk, Spanish), Watermelon, Nectarines, Papaya, Peaches, Pears, Persimmons, Pineapple, Pomegranates, Prickly pears, Raisins, Raspberries, Starfruit, Strawberries **Juices-** Apricot, Carrot, Celery, Cranberry, Cucumber, Grape, Grapefruit, Papaya, Tomato, Water & lemon

Spices/Condiments

Agar, Allspice, Almond extract, Apple butter, Anise, Arrowroot, Barley malt, Basil, Bay leaf, Bergamot, Brown rice syrup, Cardamom, Chervil, Chives, Chocolate, Coriander, Cumin, Dill, Garlic, Plain Gelatin, Honey, Horseradish, Jam/Jelly from acceptable fruit, Maple syrup, Marjoram, Mayonnaise, Mint, Miso, Molasses, Dry Mustard, Mustard, Paprika, Peppercorn, Red pepper flakes, Peppermint, Pimiento, Rice syrup, Rosemary, Saffron, Sage, Salt, Savory, Soy sauce, Spearmint, Brown and White Sugar, Tamari, Tamarind, Tapioca, Tarragon, Thyme, Vanilla, Wintergreen, Worcestershire sauce

Beverages/Herbal Teas

Beer, **Tea-** Catnip, Chamomile, Dong Quai, Elder, Ginseng, Hawthorn, Horehound, Licorice, Mullein, Raspberry leaf, Sage, Skullcap, Spearmint, Thyme, Valerian, Vervain, White birch, White oak bark, Yarrow

Blood Type O

List of avoid foods

No anabolic designation is made for avoid list

Meats/Seafood
Goose, All Pork, **Seafood-** Barracuda, Catfish, Caviar, Conch, Pickled Herring, Lox, Octopus

Eggs/Dairy
American cheese, Blue cheese, Brie, Buttermilk, Camembert, Casein, Cheddar, Colby, Cottage cheese, Cream cheese, Edam, Emmenthal, Goat milk, Gouda, Gruyere, Ice cream, Jarlsberg, Kefir, Monterey Jack, Muenster, Parmesan, Provolone, Neufchatel, Ricotta, Skim or 2% milk, String cheese, Swiss, Whole Milk, Yogurt-all varieties

Oils/Fats/Nuts/Seeds
Corn oil, Cottonseed oil, Peanut oil, Safflower oil, Brazil nuts, Cashews, Litchi, Peanuts, Peanut butter, Pistachios, Poppy seeds

Beans and Legumes
Copper, Kidney, Navy and Tamarind Beans; Domestic, Green and Red Lentils

Cereals/Bread/Grains/Pasta
Cornflakes, Cornmeal, Corn muffins, Familia, Farina, Grape nuts, Oat bran, Oatmeal, Oat bran muffins, Oat flour, Shredded wheat, Wheat bran, Wheat germ, Wheat bagels, Cream of wheat, Durum wheat, Wheat matzos, Wheat bran muffins, Whole wheat bread, Bulghur wheat flour, White and whole wheat flour, English muffins, High-protein bread, Multi-grain bread, Pumpernickel, Couscous flour, Gluten flour, Graham flour, Soba noodles, Semolina and Spinach Pasta, Seven-grain

Vegetables/Fruits
CA Avocado, Brussel Sprouts, Chinese, Red and White Cabbage, Cauliflower, White and Yellow Corn, Eggplant, Domestic and Shitake Mushrooms, Mustard Greens, Black, Greek and Spanish Olives, Red and White Potatoes, Alfalfa Sprouts, **Fruits-** Blackberries, Coconuts, Cantaloupe and Honeydew Melon, Oranges, Plantains, Rhubarb; Tangerines, **Juices-** Apple and cider, Cabbage, Orange

Spices/Condiments
Capers, Cinnamon, Cornstarch, Corn syrup; Nutmeg, Black and White Pepper, Apple cider, Red Wine and White Vinegar, Balsamic, Ketchup, Pickles- Dill, Kosher, Sweet, Sour, and Relish

Beverages
Coffee, Distilled liquor, Sodas, Black Tea

A WORD OF CAUTION

Individuals may differ in their reactions to foods listed herein. This is not a medical opinion. The information contained herein is based upon public information. The authors of this material relied on the expertise of others in compiling this information.

Because not all individuals react the same to foods that should be good or are listed as good or highly beneficial, it is a good idea to monitor those beneficial foods, which may cause some discomfort. We know because, having tried almost every food, and after following others who have adhered to the diet, we found some inconsistencies and some foods, which for one reason or another several of our test subjects could not tolerate. We found several AB's who could not tolerate grape juice or sour cherries, which are very beneficial. Because of their body chemistry these foods were too rich, or were not tolerated well.

We also found several subjects could not tolerate tofu and wine at the same sitting. It was necessary for at least an hour to pass before they had a glass of wine. Apparently, their systems just did not tolerate the mixture. Eating or drinking the foods apart caused no distress, but only your particular body chemistry, through trial and error, will provide the best combination of foods for you.

A further note of caution for As and ABs regarding the listed foods above. These two blood groups are considerably more susceptible to saturated fat in the short run. As we stated earlier, saturated fat is bad and unnecessary for all blood types, and given enough time will become a problem for Blood Types O and B, also. However, as it applies to As and ABs, we would not recommend lamb or goat's milk on a regular basis. Both lamb and goat's milk are delicious, but they are just too high in saturated animal fat, and could be a definite problem for the A and ABs.

If you do eat lamb, we suggest a glass of red wine with the meal. Red wine is listed as beneficial for ABs. The skin or pulp and the alcohol content in the wine in conjunction with any saturated fat will have the effect of preventing the absorption of part of the fat into the blood stream, thereby preventing it from depositing on artery walls. In addition, the wine should raise your HDL cholesterol level, thereby providing another preventative measure against heart disease. This is another reason we recommend one glass of red wine a day for A and ABs.

<u>CONCLUSION</u>

The researchers believe most of the foods listed in the respective food groups will work well for an overwhelming number of people within that food group. But like anything else, there are exceptions to the rule. The best test is to try to eat the recommended foods on the list, avoiding those so indicated, and monitoring your results.

You should notice a reduction in bloating and gas, and a change in your metabolism and energy levels. Usually if you eat only highly beneficial foods you will lose weight. Neutral foods are just that; they are good for you. Although you may not feel all or any of the harmful effects of the "to avoid" foods, research has shown they cause agglutination of blood, hypoglycemia, gas, bloating, improper metabolism, weight gain, lower immune function, and may contribute to a higher risk of disease.

A special note for Type As:

The foods most harmful to As in the long run are meat and dairy. The elimination of these two food groups will allow Type A individuals the greatest potential to avoid heart disease and cancer. Tofu, soy products, red skinned unsalted peanuts, red wine, and green tea are especially good for Type As, as they help fight cancer and heart disease.

A special note for Type ABs:

The single worst food for an AB is chicken. Chicken contains a dangerous lectin that may agglutinate the blood and may also lead to heart disease, cancer and/or a host of other digestive and intestinal tract illnesses. Tofu, soy products, red skinned unsalted peanuts, red wine, and green tea are especially good for Type AB as they help fight cancer and heart disease.

A special note for Type Bs:

The authors would urge Type B individuals to eliminate all wheat, corn, tomatoes, peanuts, and especially, chicken, from their diet. Chicken contains a dangerous lectin that may agglutinate the blood and may also lead to heart disease, cancer, diverticulitis, irritable bowel syndrome, spastic colon, cancer of the colon and/or a host of other digestive and intestinal tract illnesses. When our research subjects stopped eating chicken, many of their symptoms abated.

A special note for Type Os:

As healthy as Type Os appeared in our research, it is recommended that they eliminate most dairy, nuts, and grains, with the exceptions listed in the beneficial and neutral food groups. Type Os that eliminate the "avoid" dairy and grain products and stick to lean protein tend to have very low cholesterol levels and stay quite healthy.

Items not available in your local market should be available in natural or health food stores

PHYSICALLY INACTIVE PERSON
7-DAY MENU FOR TYPE A

Day 1

Breakfast:
1/2 squeezed lemon in 4 oz. of water
1/2 grapefruit or 4 oz. grapefruit juice not from concentrate
Bowl of amaranth flakes with blueberries, raisins, or blackberries
1 slice of Essene bread with apricot jelly or jam
One cup of coffee
One scoop of Personal Protein in 4 to 5 oz. of cold water, or soy milk

Lunch:
Bowl of lentil soup
Romaine Lettuce salad with carrots, onions, artichoke, alfalfa sprouts, and grilled tofu
8 oz. glass of pineapple juice

Afternoon Snack:
One large apple (provides 5 grams of fiber)
10 to 12 oz. of water or green tea

Dinner:
1/4 crenshaw melon
Small can of sockeye salmon with diced celery and onions
Black beans and white rice sprinkled with fresh garlic
Broccoli and carrots
10 to 12 oz. of green tea or glass of red wine

Evening Snack:
Tamari/Seaweed rice cakes with melted soy cheese
Glass of red wine, green tea, or soy milk

Before Bedtime:
One scoop of Personal Protein in 4 to 5 oz. of water

PHYSICALLY INACTIVE PERSON
7-DAY MENU FOR TYPE A

Day 2

Breakfast:
Medium bowl of cream of buckwheat with soy milk
4 or 5 figs
One cup of coffee
One scoop of Personal Protein in 4 to 5 oz. of water or soy milk

Lunch:
Peanut butter and jelly on Ezekiel bread
Sliced cucumbers, celery, and zucchini
5 or 6 apricots
10 to 12 oz. green tea

Afternoon Snack:
One cup black coffee**
Oat bran muffin
**Coffee should be taken black or with soy milk, no dairy milk or cream

Dinner:
Cold pumpkin soup
6 to 8 oz. fresh sliced turkey breast (not smoked), with cranberry sauce or
   dried cranberries
Large mixed salad of acceptable greens with feta cheese, and pinto beans
One 8-oz. glass of red wine or 10 to 12 oz. of water or green tea

Evening Snack:
Mixed Macadamia nuts, almonds, and raisins
10 to 12 oz. of water, green tea, or glass of red wine

Before Bedtime:
One scoop of Personal Protein in 4 to 5 oz. of cold water

PHYSICALLY INACTIVE PERSON
7-DAY MENU FOR TYPE A

Day 3

Breakfast:
Two egg omelet with onion, scallions, and chopped broccoli
One slice of toasted sprouted wheat bread with grape or strawberry jam
  or jelly
One cup coffee with soy milk
One scoop of Personal Protein with 4 to 5 oz. of cold water, or soy milk

Lunch:
Medley of raw or steamed acceptable vegetables
Assorted acceptable fruits or yogurt
10 to 12 oz. of green tea

Afternoon Snack:
Any acceptable fruit (apple, plum, figs, etc.)
10 to 12 oz. of water, or apricot juice

Dinner:
Albacore tuna with diced celery on tamari/seaweed rice cakes
Medium salad with soy cheese, garlic miso dressing
Side of green beans
One glass red wine or 10 to 12 oz. of water or green tea

Evening Snack:
Mixed Macadamia nuts and red skinned unsalted peanuts
8 to 10 oz. of green tea or glass of red wine

Before Bedtime:
One scoop of Personal Protein with 4 to 5 oz. of cold water

PHYSICALLY INACTIVE PERSON
7-DAY MENU FOR TYPE A

Day 4

Breakfast:

1/2 grapefruit or 4 oz. of pineapple, grapefruit, prune, celery, or carrot
  juice
Medium bowl cream of buckwheat with raisins
One slice Essene bread with boysenberry, blueberry, or blackberry jelly or
  jam
One cup of coffee
One scoop of Personal Protein in 4 to 5 oz. of cold water, or soy milk

Lunch:

Bowl of miso soup
Mixed green salad with sliced tempeh, grilled tofu, parsley, artichoke, with
  ginger garlic dressing
Glass of cranberry or black cherry juice, or 10 to 12 oz. of water or
  green tea

Afternoon Snack:

Small bowl of raspberries, strawberries, or loganberries
Glass of soy milk

Dinner:

8 oz. filet of grouper, snapper, or rainbow trout
Side of pinto beans with dash of soy sauce
Side of broccoli, pasta in garlic and oil, or white rice
Glass of red wine or 10 to 12 oz. of water or green tea

Evening Snack:

8 to 10 cherries, figs, or apricots, mix if preferred
10 to 12 oz. of green tea

Before Bedtime:

One scoop of Personal Protein in 4 to 5 oz. of cold water

PHYSICALLY INACTIVE PERSON
7-DAY MENU FOR TYPE A

Day 5

Breakfast:

One medium bowl of oat bran, oatmeal, puffed rice, spelt, or corn flakes, with soymilk. Mix if desired.
One slice sprouted wheat bread with acceptable jelly or jam
4 or 5 figs
Cup of coffee
One scoop of Personal Protein in 4 to 5 oz. of water

Lunch:

Artichoke pasta with garlic and olive oil
Steamed vegetables of broccoli, carrots, onions, and parsnips
10 to 12 oz. of green tea or glass of red wine

Afternoon Snack:

One oat bran muffin, or three rye crisps
10 to 12 oz. of water or green tea

Dinner:

8 oz. of chicken breast, basted in garlic, soy sauce or tamari
Mixed green salad with sprinkled goat cheese, feta cheese, or low fat mozzarella
Side of aduke or azuki beans
10 to 12 oz. of green tea or glass of red wine

Evening Snack:

Mixed peanuts, macadamia nuts, and raisins
4 to 6 oz. of pineapple or apricot juice

Before Bedtime:

One scoop of Personal Protein in 4 to 5 oz. of cold water

PHYSICALLY INACTIVE PERSON
7-DAY MENU FOR TYPE A

Day 6

Breakfast:
Medium bowl of cream of kasha with raisin and soy milk
One slice of sprouted wheat bread with jelly or jam
Two plums or 1/2 dozen apricots
One cup of coffee
One scoop of Personal Protein with 4 to 5 oz. cold water, or soy milk

Lunch:
Cold carrot soup with onions
Black beans and white rice with tamari or soy sauce
10 to 12 oz. of green tea or water

Afternoon Snack:
One large apple, two plums, or five or six figs
10 to 12 oz. of green tea or water

Dinner:
One medium Cornish hen
Mixed green salad of alfalfa sprouts, onions, grilled tofu, beet leaves, and
    dandelion with lemon dressing
Side of yellow corn
10 to 12 oz. of green tea, water, or glass of red wine

Evening Snack:
Peanut butter and jelly on toasted raisin Ezekiel bread
10 to 12 oz. of green tea, water, or soy milk

Before Bedtime:
One scoop of Personal Protein in 4 to 5 oz. of cold water

PHYSICALLY INACTIVE PERSON
7-DAY MENU FOR TYPE A

Day 7

Breakfast:
Medium bowl of amaranth flakes with raisins in soy milk
One slice Essene bread with acceptable jelly or jam
One plum, three or four figs, or six apricots
Cup of coffee
One scoop of Personal Protein in 4 to 5 oz. of water or soy milk

Lunch:
Black beans and white rice
Small green salad with garlic dill dressing
One corn muffin with blackstrap molasses
6 oz. of pineapple chunks
10 to 12 oz. of green tea

Afternoon Snack:
Mixed fruit, apricots, figs, cherries, and/or cranberries
6 oz. of pineapple or apricot juice or 10 to 12 oz. of green tea

Dinner:
6 or 8 oz. filet of mackerel, salmon, sea trout, cod, or pickerel
Side of spinach, kale, romaine lettuce, carrots, and/or alfalfa sprouts
Side of soba noodles, or rice of choice
Glass of red wine or 10 to 12 oz. of water or green tea

Evening Snack:
Mixed acceptable nuts
10 to 12 ounces of green tea (you may alternate wine with green tea as
  preferred)

Before Bedtime:
One scoop of Personal Protein in 4 to 5 oz. of cold water

**A final note regarding the Type A diet. We believe individuals of this
blood type has the most difficult diet to follow because it is so radically
different from the American diet rich is meat, potatoes and saturated
fat. This is why type As die the youngest. Meat, potatoes, and saturated
fats kill As faster because of their inherent thick blood. The above avoid
foods are inconsistent with As blood enzymes, and it is only a matter of
time before high blood pressure, diabetes, and heart disease take their
toll as the statistics indicate.**

PHYSICALLY ACTIVE PERSON
7-DAY MENU FOR TYPE A

Day 1

Breakfast:
1/2 squeezed lemon in 4 oz. of water
Bowl of amaranth flakes, with soy milk
1 slice of Essene bread with apricot jelly or jam
One cup of coffee
Two scoops of Personal Protein in 10 to 12 oz. cold water

Lunch:
6 oz. filet of chicken
Romaine Lettuce salad with feta cheese, walnuts, alfalfa sprouts, and
   grilled tofu
12 oz. glass of water or green tea

Afternoon snack:
Protein bar - 20-35 grams, or protein shake
10 to 12 oz. of water or green tea

Dinner:
Small can of sockeye salmon with diced celery and onions
Assorted cheeses, mozzarella, farmer, and string
Side green beans
10 to 12 oz. of water, green tea or glass of red wine

Evening Snack:
Toasted Ezekiel bread with melted soy cheese
Glass of red wine, green tea, or soy milk

Before Bedtime:
Two scoops of Personal Protein in 10 to 12 oz. cold water

PHYSICALLY ACTIVE PERSON
7-DAY MENU FOR TYPE A

Day 2

Breakfast:
Two eggs boiled, poached, or scrambled
3 or 4 slices of turkey bacon (this is turkey not pork)
One cup of coffee
Two scoops of Personal Protein in 10 to 12 oz. cold water

Lunch:
Peanut butter and jelly on Essene bread
10 to 12 oz. of water or green tea

Afternoon Snack:
Protein bar - 20 to 35 grams, or protein shake
10 to 12 oz. of water or green tea

Dinner:
Cold pumpkin soup
6 to 8 oz. grilled or broiled chicken breast
Large mixed salad of acceptable greens with feta cheese, grilled tofu, and
  pinto beans
One 8-oz. glass of red wine or 10 to 12 oz. of water or green tea

Evening Snack:
Mixed Macadamia, almonds, walnuts
10 to 12 oz. of water, green tea, or glass of red wine

Before Bedtime:
Two scoops of Personal Protein in 10 to 12 oz. cold water

PHYSICALLY ACTIVE PERSON
7-DAY MENU FOR TYPE A

Day 3

Breakfast:
Medium bowl of cream of buckwheat
One slice toasted sprouted wheat bread with grape or strawberry jam or jelly
One cup coffee with soy milk
Two scoops of Personal Protein with 10 to 12 oz. cold water

Lunch:
Medley of raw or steamed acceptable vegetables with grilled tofu or tempeh
10 to 12 oz. of water, or green tea

Afternoon Snack:
Protein bar - 20-35 grams, or protein shake
10 to 12 oz. of water or green tea

Dinner:
Albacore tuna with diced celery
Medium salad with soy cheese, feta cheese, garlic miso dressing
Side of aduki beans
One glass red wine or 10 to 12 oz. of water or green tea

Evening Snack:
Mixed peanuts** and Macadamia nuts
8 to 10 oz. of green tea or glass of red wine
**Peanuts should be raw from shell with brown skin

Before Bedtime:
Two scoops of Personal Protein with 10 to 12 oz. cold water

PHYSICALLY ACTIVE PERSON
7-DAY MENU FOR TYPE A

Day 4

Breakfast:
1/2 grapefruit or 3 oz. of pineapple, grapefruit, prune, celery, or carrot juice
Medium bowl amaranth flakes with soymilk
One slice Essene bread with boysenberry, blueberry, or blackberry jelly or jam
One cup of coffee
Two scoops of Personal Protein in 10 to 12 oz. cold water.

Lunch:
Bowl of miso soup
Mixed green salad with sliced tempeh, parsley, ginger garlic dressing
10 to 12 oz. of water or green tea

Afternoon Snack:
Protein bar - 20-35 grams, or protein shake
Glass of soymilk, green tea, or 12 oz. glass of water

Dinner:
8 oz. filet of grouper, snapper, or rainbow trout
Side brown, black or green soybeans (edamame) (remove outside pod before eating)
Side of broccoli or broccoli sprouts
Glass of red wine or 10 to 12 oz. of water or green tea

Evening Snack:
Mixed acceptable nuts
10 to 12 oz. of water, green tea

Before Bedtime:
Two scoops of Personal Protein in 10 to 12 oz. cold water

PHYSICALLY ACTIVE PERSON
7-DAY MENU FOR TYPE A

Day 5

Breakfast:
One medium bowl of oat bran, oatmeal, puffed rice, spelt, or cornflakes,
  with soymilk. (Mix dry cereals if desired.)
One slice sprouted wheat bread with acceptable jelly or jam
Cup of coffee
Two scoops of Personal Protein in 10 to 12 oz. cold water

Lunch:
Can of sockeye salmon or albacore tuna
Steamed vegetables of broccoli, carrots, onions, and grilled tofu
10 to 12 oz. of green tea or glass of red wine

Afternoon Snack:
Protein bar - 20-35 grams, or protein shake
10 to 12 oz. of water

Dinner:
8 oz. of chicken breast, basted in garlic, soy sauce or tamari
Mixed green salad with sprinkled goat cheese, feta cheese, or low fat
  mozzarella
Side of black, brown, or green soybeans
10 to 12 oz. of green tea or glass of red wine

Evening Snack:
Mixed peanuts and Macadamia nuts
10 to 12 oz. of green tea

Before Bedtime:
Two scoops of Personal Protein in 10 to 12 oz. cold water

PHYSICALLY ACTIVE PERSON
7-DAY MENU FOR TYPE A

Day 6

Breakfast:
Medium bowl of cream of kasha with soy milk
One slice of sprouted wheat bread with jelly or jam
One cup of coffee
Two scoops of Personal Protein with 10 to 12 oz. cold water

Lunch:
Cold carrot soup with onions
6 oz. sliced turkey breast
10 to 12 oz. of green tea or water

Afternoon Snack:
Protein bar - 20-35 grams, or protein shake
10 to 12 oz. of green tea or water

Dinner:
One medium Cornish hen
Mixed green salad of alfalfa sprouts, onions, grilled tofu, beet leaves, and
  dandelion with lemon dressing
Side of soybeans
10 to 12 oz. of green tea, water, or glass of red wine

Evening Snack:
Peanut butter and jelly on toasted raisin Ezekiel bread
10 to 12 oz. of green tea or water

Before Bedtime:
Two scoops of Personal Protein in 10 to 12 oz. cold water

PHYSICALLY ACTIVE PERSON
7-DAY MENU FOR TYPE A

Day 7

Breakfast:
Two eggs boiled, poached, or scrambled
3 or 4 slices turkey bacon
One slice Essene bread with acceptable jelly or jam
Cup of coffee
Two scoops of Personal Protein in 10 to 12 oz. cold water

Lunch:
Green salad with feta cheese, tempeh or grilled tofu with garlic dill dressing
10 to 12 oz. of water or green tea

Afternoon Snack:
Protein bar - 20-35 grams, or protein shake
10 to 12 oz. of green tea

Dinner:
6 or 8 oz. filet of mackerel, salmon, sea trout, cod, or pickerel
Side of spinach, kale, romaine lettuce, carrots, and/or alfalfa sprouts
Side of soybeans (black, brown, or green)
Glass of red wine or 10 to 12 oz. of water or green tea

Evening Snack:
Mixed acceptable nuts or peanut butter and jelly on Ezekiel bread
10 to 12 ounces of green tea (you may alternate wine with green tea as preferred)

Before Bedtime:
Two scoops of Personal Protein in 10 to 12 oz. cold water
Look for all of these items at your favorite health food store

Personal Protein available on web site 4blood.com or 1-888-41BLOOD.

PHYSICALLY INACTIVE PERSON
7-DAY MENU FOR TYPE B

Day 1

Breakfast:
6 oz. of pineapple juice
Medium bowl of oatmeal with skim milk
One banana
One slice of Ezekiel bread with butter, jelly or jam (no margarine)
Coffee, tea, water, or skim milk
One scoop of Personal Protein in 4 to 5 oz. of water or skim milk

Lunch:
Mixed green salad sprinkled with feta cheese or mozzarella (no tomato)
  and garlic/ginger dressing
Fruit yogurt
10 to 12 oz. of water or green tea

Afternoon Snack:
Bunch of grapes, cranberries, or one large apple
Coffee, tea, water, or skim milk

Dinner:
6 to 8 oz. salmon filet in lemon butter
Side of kidney beans
Side of broccoli, cauliflower, or carrots
10 to 12 oz. of water or green tea

Evening Snack:
Rice cake with apple butter, jelly or jam
10 to 12 oz. of water or green tea

Before Bedtime:
One scoop of Personal Protein in 4 to 5 oz. of cold water

PHYSICALLY INACTIVE PERSON
7-DAY MENU FOR TYPE B

Day 2

Breakfast:
6 oz. of cranberry juice
Mixed cereal of rice bran and spelt with skim milk and blueberries
One slice of Essene bread with cream cheese
Coffee, tea, water, or skim milk
One scoop of Personal Protein in 4 to 5 oz. of cold water, or skim milk

Lunch:
6-oz. fresh sliced turkey breast croissant with cranberry spread
Side of mashed potatoes
Side of cole slaw or collard greens
One pickle of choice
10 to 12 oz. of water or green tea

Afternoon Snack:
Oat bran muffin
Coffee, green tea, water, or skim milk

Dinner:
8 oz. lean ground beef with Worcestershire sauce (no ketchup)
Mixed green salad with goat cheese and olive oil and lemon dressing
Side of sweet potato
Side of kale
10 to 12 oz. of green tea, water, or glass of red or white wine

Evening Snack:
Grilled cheese on toasted raisin Ezekiel bread
Coffee, green tea, water, or skim milk

Before Bedtime:
One scoop of Personal Protein in 4 to 5 oz. of cold water

PHYSICALLY INACTIVE PERSON
7-DAY MENU FOR TYPE B

Day 3

Breakfast:
4 oz. glass of papaya juice
Two eggs boiled, poached, or scrambled
Side of hashed brown potatoes or garlic roasted red potatoes
One slice of toasted millet bread with butter, jelly, or jam
Coffee, tea, water, or skim milk
One scoop of Personal Protein in 4 to 5 oz. of cold water, or skim milk

Lunch:
6 oz. filet of cod or haddock (grilled or baked)
Side of lima beans
Side of Brussels sprouts
10 to 12 oz. of green tea or water

Afternoon Snack:
One large apple or banana
Coffee, green tea, water, or skim milk

Dinner:
Pasta with sautéed scallops and pea pods, in garlic and olive oil
Mixed green salad with carrots, beets, parsley, and green and yellow peppers/balsamic vinegar
Italian bread with melted mozzarella, parmesan, provolone or acceptable cheese
One or two glasses of white wine

Evening Snack:
Grilled cheese on toasted Ezekiel bread
Coffee, tea, water, or skim milk

Before Bedtime:
One scoop of Personal Protein in 4 to 5 oz. of cold water

PHYSICALLY INACTIVE PERSON
7-DAY MENU FOR TYPE B

Day 4

Breakfast:
4 oz. of grape juice
Medium bowl of cream of rice with acceptable fruit
One slice of fin crisp with jelly or jam
Coffee, tea, water, or skim milk
One scoop of Personal Protein in 4 to 5 oz. of cold water or skim milk

Lunch:
Bowl of navy bean soup (no pork or ham); use acceptable spices for additional flavor
Albacore tuna cheese melt, with celery, onions, and mayonnaise
Side of sliced cucumbers, mustard greens, or broccoli
10 to 12 oz. of water or green tea

Afternoon Snack:
Assorted fruits (apple, apricots, figs)
Coffee, tea, water, or skim milk

Dinner:
Grilled liver and onions
Side of broccoli, shitake mushrooms, kale or beets
Mixed lettuce salad with farmer cheese and kidney beans
10 to 12 oz. of green tea, water, or glass of red or white wine

Evening Snack:
Rice cakes with almond butter
Coffee, green tea, water, or skim milk

Before Bedtime:
One scoop of Personal Protein in 4 to 5 oz. of cold water

PHYSICALLY INACTIVE PERSON
7-DAY MENU FOR TYPE B

Day 5

Breakfast:
6 oz. of pineapple juice
Medium bowl of oatmeal with acceptable fruit
One slice of wasa bread with butter, jelly or jam
Coffee, tea, water, or skim milk
One scoop of Personal Protein in 4 to 5 oz. of cold water, or skim milk

Lunch:
Fruit yogurt
Mixed green salad with cheese of choice and low fat dressing
10 to 12 oz. of water or green tea

Afternoon Snack:
Vegetable cocktail or fruit cocktail from acceptable fruits and vegetables

Dinner:
8 oz. filet mignon in lemon butter
One sweet potato with cinnamon butter or baked potato with butter, yogurt or sour cream
Mixed green salad of onions, scallions, mushrooms, asparagus, garlic, and endive
10 to 12 oz. of green tea, water, or glass of red or white wine

Evening Snack:
Grilled cheese on toasted raisin Ezekiel bread.
Coffee, tea, water or skim milk

Before Bedtime:
One scoop of Personal Protein in 4 to 5 oz. of cold water

PHYSICALLY INACTIVE PERSON
7-DAY MENU FOR TYPE B

Day 6

Breakfast:

4 oz. of pineapple juice
Mixed cereal of millet, puffed rice, and spelt with banana
One slice of toasted brown rice bread with cream cheese
Cup of coffee, tea, water, or skim milk
One scoop of Personal Protein in 4 to 5 oz. of cold water, or skim milk

Lunch:

6 oz. of sturgeon
3 oz. of caviar with onions
One or two slices of fin crisp or wasa bread (for caviar)
10 to 12 oz. of green tea or water

Dinner:

6 oz. of flank streak or fresh sliced turkey breast
Side of broccoli
Side of yams or sweet potato
Side of kidney beans
10 to 12 oz. of green tea, water, or glass of red wine

Evening Snack:

Grilled soy cheese sandwich on toasted raisin Ezekiel bread
10 to 12 oz. of green tea, water, or glass of red wine

Before Bedtime:

One scoop of Personal Protein in 4 to 5 oz. of cold water

PHYSICALLY INACTIVE PERSON
7-DAY MENU FOR TYPE B

Day 7

Breakfast:
4 oz. of cranberry juice
Two eggs boiled, poached, or scrambled
Three slices turkey bacon (this is a turkey product/not a pork product)
One slice of toasted brown rice bread with butter, jelly, or jam
Cup of coffee, tea, water, or skim milk

Lunch:
Cabbage soup with cayenne pepper and parsley
Plain or fruit yogurt
Two or three fin crisps or wasa bread with butter, jelly or jam
10 to 12 oz. of green tea or water

Afternoon Snack:
Oat bran muffin
Coffee, green tea, water, or skim milk

Dinner:
White pizza (no tomato sauce) with mozzarella, ricotta, parmesan or pro-
    volone
Mixed green salad of lettuce, carrots, broccoli, beats and lima beans, olive
    oil & balsamic vinegar
10 to 12 oz. of green tea, water, or glass of red wine

Evening Snack:
Mixed almonds and Macadamia nuts
Coffee, green tea, water, or skim milk

Before Bedtime:
One scoop of Personal Protein in 4 to 5 oz. of water

Personal Protein available on web site 4blood.com or 1-888-41BLOOD.

PHYSICALLY ACTIVE PERSON
7-DAY MENU FOR TYPE B

Day 1

Breakfast:
Medium bowl of oatmeal with skim milk
One banana
One slice of Ezekiel bread with butter (no margarine)
Coffee, green tea, water, or skim milk
Two scoops of Personal Protein in 10 to 12 oz. cold water

Lunch:
Mixed green salad sprinkled with feta cheese or mozzarella (no tomato)
   and garlic/ginger dressing
10 to 12 oz. of water or green tea

Afternoon Snack:
Protein bar - 20-35 grams, or protein shake
10 to 12 oz. of green tea, water, or skim milk

Dinner:
6 to 8 oz. salmon filet in lemon butter
Side of kidney beans
Side of broccoli, cauliflower, or carrots
10 to 12 oz. of water or green tea

Evening Snack:
Assorted beneficial cheeses
10 to 12 oz. of water or green tea

Before Bedtime:
Two scoops of Personal Protein in 10 to 12 oz. cold water

PHYSICALLY ACTIVE PERSON
7-DAY MENU FOR TYPE B

Day 2

Breakfast:
Mixed cereal of rice bran and spelt with skim milk and blueberries
One slice of Essene bread with cream cheese
Coffee, green tea, water, or skim milk
Two scoops of Personal Protein in 10 to 12 oz. of cold water

Lunch:
6 oz. fresh sliced turkey breast
Side salad of greens, and mixed beneficial cheeses
Side of cole slaw or collard greens
One pickle of choice
10 to 12 oz. of water or green tea

Afternoon Snack:
Protein bar - 20-35 grams, or protein shake
10 to 12 oz. of water or green tea

Dinner:
8 oz. lean ground beef with Worcestershire sauce (no ketchup)
Mixed green salad with goat cheese and olive oil and lemon dressing
Side of sweet potato
10 to 12 oz. of green tea, water, or glass of red or white wine

Evening Snack:
Grilled cheese on toasted raisin Ezekiel bread
10 to 12 oz. of water or green tea

Before Bedtime:
Two scoops of Personal Protein in 10 to 12 oz. cold water

PHYSICALLY ACTIVE PERSON
7-DAY MENU FOR TYPE B

Day 3

Breakfast:

Two eggs boiled, poached, or scrambled
3 or 4 slices of turkey bacon
One slice of toasted millet bread with butter
Coffee, green tea, water, or skim milk
Two scoops of Personal Protein in 10 to 12 oz. cold water

Lunch:

6 oz. filet of cod or haddock (grilled or baked)
Side of lima beans
Two or three slices of acceptable beneficial/assorted cheeses
10 to 12 oz. of green tea or water

Afternoon Snack:

Protein bar - 20-35 grams, or protein shake
10 to 12 oz. of water or green tea

Dinner:

Sautéed scallops and pea pods, in garlic and olive oil
Mixed green salad with carrots, beets, parsley, feta cheese/balsamic vinegar dressing
10 to 12 oz. of water or green tea

Evening Snack:

Grilled cheese on toasted Ezekiel bread
10 to 12 oz. of water or green tea

Before Bedtime:

Two scoops of Personal Protein in 10 to 12 oz. cold water

PHYSICALLY ACTIVE PERSON
7-DAY MENU FOR TYPE B

Day 4

Breakfast:

Two eggs boiled, poached, or scrambled
3 or 4 slices of turkey bacon
One slice of fin crisp with jelly or jam
Coffee, green tea, water, or skim milk
Two scoops of Personal Protein in 10 to 12 oz. cold water or skim milk

Lunch:

Bowl of navy bean soup (no pork or ham); use acceptable spices for additional flavor
Albacore tuna cheese melt, with celery, onions, and mayonnaise
10 to 12 oz. of water or green tea

Afternoon Snack:

Protein bar - 20-35 grams, or protein shake
10 -12 oz. of water or green tea

Dinner:

Grilled liver and onions
Side of broccoli, shitake mushrooms, kale or beets
Mixed lettuce salad with farmer cheese and kidney beans
10 to 12 oz. of green tea, water, or glass of red or white wine

Evening Snack:

Assorted beneficial and/or neutral cheeses, or Macadamia nuts
10- 12 oz. of water or green tea

Before Bedtime:

Two scoops of Personal Protein in 10 to 12 oz. cold water

PHYSICALLY ACTIVE PERSON
7-DAY MENU FOR TYPE B

Day 5

Breakfast:
3 oz. of pineapple juice
Medium bowl of oatmeal
One slice of wasa bread with butter
Coffee, green tea, water, or skim milk
Two scoops of Personal Protein in 10 to12 oz. cold water

Lunch:
Sliced turkey breast
Mixed green salad with cheese and beans of choice, acceptable dressing
10 to 12 oz. of water or green tea

Afternoon Snack:
Protein bar - 20-35 grams, or protein shake
10 to 12 oz. of water or green tea

Dinner:
8 oz. filet mignon in lemon butter
One sweet potato or baked potato with butter
Mixed green salad of onions, scallions, mushrooms, asparagus, garlic, and
  Swiss cheese
10 to 12 oz. of green tea, water, or glass of red or white wine

Evening Snack:
Grilled cheese of choice on toasted raisin Ezekiel bread.
10 to 12 oz. of water or green tea

Before Bedtime:
Two scoops of Personal Protein in 10 to 12 oz. cold water

PHYSICALLY ACTIVE PERSON
7-DAY MENU FOR TYPE B

Day 6

Breakfast:
Mixed cereal of millet, puffed rice, and spelt with banana
One slice of toasted brown rice bread with cream cheese
Cup of coffee, green tea, water, or skim milk
Two scoops of Personal Protein in 10 to 12 oz. cold water

Lunch:
6 oz. of sturgeon
3 oz. of caviar with onions on fin or wasa bread
10 to 12 oz. of water or green tea

Afternoon Snack:
Protein bar - 20-35 grams, or protein shake
10 to 12 oz. of water or green tea

Dinner:
6 oz. of flank streak or fresh sliced turkey breast
Mixed green salad with kidney beans and cheese of choice, dressing
  of choice
10 to 12 oz. of green tea, water, or glass of red wine

Evening Snack:
Grilled Mozzarella cheese sandwich on toasted raisin Ezekiel bread
10 to 12 oz. of green tea, water, or glass of red wine

Before Bedtime:
Two scoops of Personal Protein in 10 to 12 oz. cold water

PHYSICALLY ACTIVE PERSON
7-DAY MENU FOR TYPE B

Day 7

Breakfast:
3 oz. glass of papaya juice
Two eggs boiled, poached, or scrambled
Three slices turkey bacon (this is a turkey product/not a pork product)
One slice of toasted brown rice bread with butter
Two scoops of Personal Protein in 10 to 12 oz. cold water

Lunch:
6 oz. hamburger with melted Swiss or Mozzarella/ no bread
1 medium baked potato with butter
10 to 12 oz. of green tea or water

Afternoon Snack:
Protein bar - 20-35 grams, or protein shake
10 to 12 oz. of water or green tea

Dinner:
White pizza (no tomato sauce) with mozzarella, ricotta, parmesan or provolone
Mixed green salad of lettuce, carrots, broccoli sprouts, beats and lima
beans, olive oil & balsamic vinegar
10 to 12 oz. of green tea, water, or glass of red wine

Evening Snack:
Mixed almonds and Macadamia nuts
10 to 12 oz. of coffee, green tea, or water

Before Bedtime:
Two scoops of Personal Protein in 10 to 12 oz. cold water
Look for all of these items at your favorite health food store

Personal Protein available on web site 4blood.com or 1-888-41BLOOD.

PHYSICALLY INACTIVE PERSON
7-DAY MENU FOR TYPE AB

Day 1

Breakfast:
1/2 squeezed lemon in 4 oz. of water
1/2 grapefruit or 4 oz. of grapefruit juice (not from concentrate)
One kiwi, or bunch of seedless grapes (20 - 30 grapes)
Medium bowl of oatmeal with rice milk
One slice of Ezekiel bread with acceptable jelly or jam (without corn syrup)
One cup of coffee (skim milk is optional)
One scoop of Personal Protein in 4 to 5 oz. of cold water, or rice milk

Lunch:
6 oz. of fresh sliced turkey breast (not smoked)
Small portion of cranberries or cranberry sauce
Side order of non-fat cottage cheese
Side of sliced cucumbers or broccoli
10 to 12 oz. of green tea

Afternoon Snack:
One large apple (provides 5 grams of fiber)
10 to 12 oz. of water, green tea, or cup of coffee

Dinner:
Albacore tuna with celery, onions, and fat free mayonnaise
One or two rice cakes of choice (tamari & seaweed)
Mixed green salad of acceptable greens with sliced grilled tofu, feta
  cheese, and garlic miso dressing
Glass of red wine or 10 to 12 oz. of water or green tea

Evening Snack:
Mixed roasted red-skinned peanuts and Macadamia nuts
10 to 12 oz. of water or green tea or glass of red wine

Before Bedtime:
One scoop of Personal Protein in 4 to 5 oz. of cold water

PHYSICALLY INACTIVE PERSON
7-DAY MENU FOR TYPE AB

Day 2

Breakfast:
Lemon water & grapefruit juice apply (you may substitute 1/2 grapefruit
    for juice)
One plum or 3 or 4 figs
One medium bowl of cream of rye (100% rye) with rice milk
One slice of Essene bread with acceptable jelly or jam
One cup of coffee
One scoop of Personal Protein in 4 to 5 oz. of cold water

Lunch:
Mixed green salad, sliced tomatoes, one square cut grilled tofu, olive oil,
    lemon juice and acceptable spices
One plain or fruit yogurt from acceptable fruit
10 to 12 oz. of water or green tea

Afternoon Snack:
Cup of coffee
Oat bran muffin

Dinner:
6 to 8 oz. filet of Salmon with squeezed lemon
One medium sweet potato
1/2 cup navy beans
10 to 12 oz. of water, green tea, or glass of red wine

Evening Snack:
Peanut butter and jelly on toasted Ezekiel bread
10 to 12 oz. of water or green tea (glass of red wine if not taken at dinner)

Before Bedtime:
One scoop of Personal Protein in 4 to 5 oz. of cold water

PHYSICALLY INACTIVE PERSON
7-DAY MENU FOR TYPE AB

Day 3

Breakfast:
4 oz. of pineapple chunks
One medium bowl of mixed cereal (We suggest mixing spelt, puffed rice &
  millet), with raisins and rice milk or soy milk
One slice of sprouted wheat bread with jelly or jam
One cup of coffee
One scoop of Personal Protein in 4 to 5 oz. of cold water

Lunch:
Side order of semolina pasta, in garlic and olive oil
Mixed green salad with goat cheese, mozzarella, or feta cheese, squeezed
  lemon dressing and acceptable spices
10 to 12 oz. of water or green tea

Afternoon Snack:
A bunch of seedless grapes, cherries, or five or six apricots
Cup of coffee or 10 or 12 oz. of water or green tea

Dinner:
Cold cucumber soup
Grilled or broiled lamb chops with mint jelly
One medium baked or mashed potato
Side of broccoli
Glass of red wine

Evening Snack:
Peanut butter and jelly on rice cake
10 to 12 oz. of water or green tea

Before Bedtime:
One scoop of Personal Protein in 4 to 5 oz. of cold water

PHYSICALLY INACTIVE PERSON
7-DAY MENU FOR TYPE AB

Day 4

Breakfast:
4 oz. papaya juice
Two eggs boiled, poached, or scrambled
One slice toasted sprouted wheat bread with jelly or jam
One cup coffee
One scoop of Personal Protein in 4 to 5 oz. cold water

Lunch:
Cup or bowl of green lentil soup
Side order of rice of your choice
Mixed green salad with celery, cucumber, parsley, tofu, beets, onions, scallions, garlic & oil dressing
10 to 12 oz. of water or green tea

Afternoon Snack:
One large apple, oat bran muffin, or 6 oz. of pineapple chunks
10 to 12 oz. of water or green tea

Dinner:
8 oz. filet of red snapper, mahi-mahi, or grouper
Side of red beans
Side of broccoli or cauliflower
Side of alfalfa sprouts
Glass of red wine or 10 to 12 oz. of water or green tea

Evening Snack:
Peanut butter and jelly on toasted Ezekiel bread, sprouted wheat, or Essene bread
10 to 12 oz. of water or green tea or glass of red wine

Before Bedtime:
One scoop of Personal Protein in 4 to 5 oz. of cold water

PHYSICALLY INACTIVE PERSON
7-DAY MENU FOR TYPE AB

Day 5

Breakfast:
1/2 grapefruit, 2 oz. of papaya or grape juice
One plum or 4 or 5 figs
Medium bowl of oatmeal with raisins, skim milk, rice milk, or soy milk
One slice of brown rice bread, 100% rye bread, or soy flour bread with jelly or jam
One cup of coffee
One scoop of Personal Protein in 4 to 5 oz. of water

Lunch:
1/4 Crenshaw, honeydew, cantaloupe, or acceptable melon
Small can sockeye salmon with no fat mayonnaise, celery, and onions
Small mixed green salad with pinto beans, feta cheese, garlic and lemon dressing
10 to 12 oz. of water or green tea

Afternoon Snack:
Fruit yogurt from acceptable fruit
10 to 12 oz. of water or green tea

Dinner:
Miso soup
Grilled or cold tofu
Side order of green soy beans (edamame)
Side order of white or brown rice
Tuna or salmon sashimi (raw), or seared (tataki), or broiled
10 to 12 oz. of green tea

Evening Snack:
Raw peanuts with skins with Macadamia nuts
10 to 12 oz. of water, green tea, or glass of red wine

Before Bedtime:
One scoop of Personal Protein in 4 to 5 oz. of water

PHYSICALLY INACTIVE PERSON
7-DAY MENU FOR TYPE AB

Day 6

Breakfast:
Mixed cereal of puffed rice, millet, spelt, with raisins and rice milk
One slice of toasted sprouted wheat bread with jelly or jam
20 to 30 grapes
One cup of coffee
One scoop of Personal Protein in 4 to 5 oz. of cold water

Lunch:
Red beans and rice in garlic miso dressing
Side of broccoli or tomatoes
10 to 12 oz. of water or green tea

Afternoon Snack:
One large apple or oat bran muffin
One cup of coffee

Dinner:
Individual or Medium size pizza (mozzarella, ricotta, or soy cheese/most
   have mozzarella)
Mixed green salad with tofu, celery, cucumbers, olive oil and lemon dressing
12 oz. of water or green tea or glass of red wine

Evening Snack:
1/2 dozen walnuts or raw peanuts
12 oz. of water, green tea, or glass of red wine

Before Bedtime:
One scoop of Personal Protein in 4 to 5 oz. of cold water

PHYSICALLY INACTIVE PERSON
7-DAY MENU FOR TYPE AB

Day 7

Breakfast:
Medium bowl of rice bran with raisin/cranberries with rice milk
1/2 grapefruit
One plum or 4 or 5 figs
One cup of coffee
One scoop of Personal Protein in 4 to 5 oz. of cold water

Lunch:
6 oz. of Kefir or one plain yogurt
Peanut butter and jelly on sprouted wheat, Ezekiel, or Essene bread
10 to 12 oz. of water or green tea

Afternoon Snack:
Grapes, apple slices, dates, strawberries
Two or three slices of Monterey Jack, cheddar, Colby, Gouda, Swiss, or soy
   cheese
10 to 12 oz. of water or green tea

Dinner:
Grilled swordfish, scallops, or cod
Mixed green salad with tomatoes, onions, scallions, celery, dandelion,
   tofu, garlic and lemon dressing
One medium size sweet potato
Side of broccoli, cauliflower, kale, or mustard greens
One glass of red wine or 10 to 12 oz. of water or green tea

Evening Snack:
Raw peanuts with skins and Macadamia nuts
10 to 12 oz. of water or green tea

Before Bedtime:
One scoop of Personal Protein in 4 to 5 oz. cold water

Personal Protein available on web site 4blood.com or 1-888-41BLOOD.

Note: The AB menu, as you have probably noticed, has lots of grains, green tea, peanuts and peanut butter. ABs tolerate grains very well, as they are high in fiber and don't cause heart disease or cancer. Green tea is an excellent antioxidant that prevents, slows, or stops free radicals, which in turn reduces the risk of heart disease and cancer. Peanuts and organic peanut butter, while they do have fat, most is unsaturated, they are high in niacin and resveratrol, which reduce cholesterol levels, and prevent clots from forming in the blood.

PHYSICALLY ACTIVE PERSON
7-DAY MENU FOR TYPE AB

Day 1

Breakfast:
1/2 squeezed lemon in 4 oz. of water
1/2 grapefruit or 4 oz. of grapefruit juice (not from concentrate)
Medium bowl of oatmeal with rice milk
One slice of Ezekiel bread with acceptable jelly or jam (without corn syrup)
One cup of coffee (skim or soy milk optional)
Two scoops of Personal Protein in 10 to 12 oz. cold water.

Lunch:
6 oz. of fresh sliced turkey breast (not smoked)
Side order cottage cheese
Side of sliced cucumbers or broccoli
10 to 12 oz. of green tea

Afternoon Snack:
Protein bar - 20-35 grams, or protein shake
10 to 12 oz. of water or green tea

Dinner:
Albacore tuna with celery, onions, and fat free mayonnaise
Mixed green salad of acceptable greens with sliced grilled tofu, feta
  cheese, and garlic miso dressing
Side of brown-soy beans
Glass of red wine or 10 to 12 oz. of water or green tea

Evening Snack:
Mixed roasted red-skinned peanuts and Macadamia nuts
10 to 12 oz. of water or green tea or glass of red wine

Before Bedtime:
Two scoops of Personal Protein in 10 to 12 oz. cold water.

PHYSICALLY ACTIVE PERSON
7-DAY MENU FOR TYPE AB

Day 2

Breakfast:
Lemon water & grapefruit juice apply (you may substitute 1/2 grapefruit
  for juice)
One plum or 3 or 4 figs
One medium bowl of cream of rye (100% rye) with rice milk
One slice of Essene bread with acceptable jelly or jam
One cup of coffee
Two scoops of Personal Protein in 10 to 12 oz. cold water.

Lunch:
Tuna salad on mixed greens with grilled tofu, olive oil and lemon juice
One plain or fruit yogurt from acceptable fruit
10 to 12 oz. of water or green tea

Afternoon Snack:
Protein bar - 20 to 35 grams, or protein shake
10 to 12 oz. of water or green tea

Dinner:
6 to 8 oz. filet of Salmon with squeezed lemon
One medium sweet potato
1/2 cup green soy beans
10 to 12 oz. of water, green tea, or glass of red wine

Evening Snack:
Peanut butter and jelly on toasted Ezekiel bread
10 to 12 oz. of water or green tea (glass of red wine if not taken at dinner)

Before Bedtime:
Two scoops of Personal Protein in 10 to 12 oz. cold water.

PHYSICALLY ACTIVE PERSON
7-DAY MENU FOR TYPE AB

Day 3

Breakfast:
4 oz. of pineapple chunks
One medium bowl of mixed cereal (We suggest mixing spelt, puffed rice &
   millet), with rice milk
One slice of sprouted wheat bread with jelly or jam
One cup of coffee
Two scoops of Personal Protein in 10 to 12 oz. cold water.

Lunch:
Egg salad with onions, celery, and mayonnaise
Mixed green salad with goat cheese, mozzarella, or feta cheese,
   acceptable dressing
10 to 12 oz. of water or green tea

Afternoon Snack:
Protein bar - 20 to 35 grams, or protein shake
10 or 12 oz. of water or green tea

Dinner:
Cheddar cheese & mozzarella appetizer
Grilled or broiled lamb chops with mint jelly
One medium baked or mashed potato
Side of broccoli sprouts and mixed black soybeans
Glass of red wine or 10 to 12 oz. of water or green tea

Evening Snack:
Peanut butter and jelly on Essene bread
10 to 12 oz. of water or green tea

Before Bedtime:
Two scoops of Personal Protein in 10 to 12 oz. cold water.

PHYSICALLY ACTIVE PERSON
7-DAY MENU FOR TYPE AB

Day 4

Breakfast:
4 oz. papaya juice
Two eggs boiled, poached, or scrambled
One slice toasted sprouted wheat bread with jelly or jam
One cup coffee
Two scoops of Personal Protein in 10 to 12 oz. cold water.

Lunch:
Cup or bowl of green lentil soup
Mixed green salad with celery, Swiss cheese tofu, onions, soybeans, garlic & olive oil
10 to 12 oz. of water or green tea

Afternoon Snack:
Protein bar - 20 to 35 grams, or protein shake
10 to 12 oz. of water or green tea

Dinner:
8 oz. filet of red snapper, mahi-mahi, or grouper
Mixed green salad, broccoli sprouts, alfalfa sprouts, sliced tempeh, and farmer cheese
Glass of red wine or 10 to 12 oz. of water or green tea

Evening Snack:
Peanut butter and jelly on toasted Ezekiel bread, sprouted wheat, or Essene bread
10 to 12 oz. of water or green tea

Before Bedtime:
Two scoops of Personal Protein in 10 to 12 oz. cold water.

PHYSICALLY ACTIVE PERSON
7-DAY MENU FOR TYPE AB

Day 5

Breakfast:
1/2 grapefruit, 3 oz. of papaya or grape juice
One plum or 4 or 5 figs
Medium bowl of oatmeal with rice milk
One slice of brown rice bread, 100% rye bread, or soy flour bread with jelly
    or jam
One cup of coffee
Two scoops of Personal Protein in 10 to 12 oz. cold water.

Lunch:
Small can sockeye salmon with mayonnaise, celery, and onions
Small mixed green salad with pinto beans, feta cheese, grilled tofu,
    garlic & olive oil
10 to 12 oz. of water or green tea

Afternoon Snack:
Protein bar - 20 to 35 grams, or protein shake
10 to 12 oz. of water or green tea

Dinner:
Miso soup
Tuna or salmon sashimi (raw fish) grill or broil if desired
Side order of green soy beans (edamame)
Side order of white or brown rice
10 to 12 oz. of green tea

Evening Snack:
Raw peanuts with skins with Macadamia nuts
10 to 12 oz. of water, green tea, or glass of red wine

Before Bedtime:
Two scoops of Personal Protein in 10 to 12 oz. cold water.

PHYSICALLY ACTIVE PERSON
7-DAY MENU FOR TYPE AB

Day 6

Breakfast:
Two eggs boiled, poached, or scrambled
3 or 4 slices of turkey bacon
One slice of toasted sprouted wheat bread with jelly or jam
One cup of coffee
Two scoops of Personal Protein in 10 to 12 oz. cold water.

Lunch:
Tuna salad with celery, onions, and mayonnaise
Assorted cheeses, goat, cheddar, feta, and farmer
Side of broccoli sprouts and tomatoes
10 to 12 oz. of water or green tea

Afternoon Snack:
Protein bar - 20 to 35 grams, or protein shake
10 to 12 oz. of water or green tea

Dinner:
Individual or Medium size pizza (mozzarella, ricotta, or soy cheese/most
   have mozzarella)
Mixed green salad with tofu, celery, cucumbers, olive oil and lemon dressing
12 oz. water or green tea or glass of red wine
Evening Snack:
Mixed walnuts, peanuts, and Macadamia nuts
10 to 12 oz. of water or green tea

Before Bedtime:
Two scoops of Personal Protein in 10 to 12 oz. cold water.

PHYSICALLY ACTIVE PERSON
7-DAY MENU FOR TYPE AB

Day 7

Breakfast:
1/2 grapefruit
Medium bowl of oat or rice bran with skim, soy, or rice milk
One plum or 4 or 5 figs
One cup of coffee
Two scoops of Personal Protein in 10 to 12 oz. cold water.

Lunch:
Peanut butter and jelly on sprouted wheat, Ezekiel, or Essene bread
Assorted acceptable cheeses
10 to 12 oz. of water or green tea

Afternoon Snack:
Protein bar - 20 to 35 grams, or protein shake
10 to 12 oz. of water or green tea
10 to 12 oz. of water or green tea

Dinner:
Grilled swordfish, scallops, or cod
Mixed green salad with broccoli sprouts, scallions, dandelion, tofu, garlic
   and olive oil
One medium size sweet potato
One glass of red wine or 10 to 12 oz. of water or green tea

Evening Snack:
Roasted red-skinned peanuts with Macadamia nuts
10 to 12 oz. of water or green tea

Before Bedtime:
Two scoops of Personal Protein in 10 to 12 oz. cold water.
Look for all of these items at your favorite health food store

Personal Protein available on web site 4blood.com or 1-888-41BLOOD.

PHYSICALLY INACTIVE PERSON
7-DAY MENU FOR TYPE O

Day 1

Breakfast:
4 oz. of pineapple juice
One slice of toasted raisin Ezekiel bread with jelly or jam
Mixed cereal of millet, puffed rice, and spelt with soy milk
Cup of hot peppermint herbal tea
One scoop of Personal Protein in 4 to 5 oz. of cold water

Lunch:
6 oz. of fresh sliced turkey breast with cranberry spread
Romaine lettuce with garlic and onions
Two or three artichokes
10 to 12 oz. of club soda, seltzer, water, or green tea

Afternoon Snack:
Figs and prunes, or carob chip cookies with walnuts
10 to 12 oz. of club soda, water, or green tea

Dinner:
8 oz. filet mignon in lemon butter
Side of broccoli
One sweet potato
Side of sliced red peppers
10 to 12 oz. of club soda, water, green tea, or glass of red wine

Evening Snack:
Macadamia nuts and walnuts
10 to 12 oz. of club soda, water, green tea, or soy milk

Before Bedtime:
One scoop of Personal Protein in 4 to 5 oz. of cold water

PHYSICALLY INACTIVE PERSON
7-DAY MENU FOR TYPE O

Day 2

Breakfast:
4 oz. of prune juice
3 or 4 fresh or dried figs
Medium bowl of rice bran or cream of rice
One slice of Essene bread with butter, jelly or jam
Cup of hot rosehips herbal tea
One scoop of Personal Protein in to 5 oz. of cold water or soy milk

Lunch:
Small can of sockeye salmon with celery, onions, mayonnaise & cayenne
   pepper
Small mixed salad of romaine lettuce, broccoli sprouts, leeks, seaweed,
   and parsley
Glass of black cherry juice, green tea, or 10 to 12 oz. of club soda or water

Afternoon Snack:
One large apple or two plums
10 to 12 oz. of club soda, water, or green tea

Dinner:
8 oz. chicken breast in tarragon sauce
Side of spinach
Side of pinto beans with onions
Side of sliced red bell peppers with garlic dill dressing
10 to 12 oz. of club soda, green tea, water, or glass of white wine

Evening Snack:
Mixed pumpkin seeds and walnuts
10 to 12 oz. of club soda, green tea, or water

Before Bedtime:
One scoop of Personal Protein in 4 to 5 oz. of cold water

PHYSICALLY INACTIVE PERSON
7-DAY MENU FOR TYPE O

Day 3

Breakfast:
4 oz. of grape juice
Medium bowl of cream of buckwheat
One slice of toasted raisin Ezekiel bread with butter, jelly, or jam
Cup hot mulberry herbal tea
One scoop of Personal Protein in to 5 oz. of cold water or soy milk

Lunch:
Cold pumpkin soup
White rice and black-eyed peas
Side of zucchini, watercress, cucumber, and endive with garlic lemon
   dressing
10 to 12 oz. club soda, green tea, or water

Afternoon Snack:
Soy milk over blueberries, cherries, or peaches

Dinner:
Grilled or broiled 8 oz. flank steak
One medium sweet potato
Side of broccoli or broccoli sprouts
One portobello mushroom with garlic and olive oil
10 to 12 oz. of club soda, green tea, water, or glass of red wine

Evening Snack:
Soy flour bread with tahini (sesame butter or apple butter)
10 to 12 oz. of club soda, green tea, or water

Before Bedtime:
One scoop of Personal Protein in 4 to 5 oz. of cold water

PHYSICALLY INACTIVE PERSON
7-DAY MENU FOR TYPE O

Day 4

Breakfast:
4 oz. of apricot juice
Two eggs any style
Three strips of turkey bacon (this is turkey, not pork)
One slice of Essene bread with butter, apple butter, jelly or jam
Cup of hot Sarsaparilla herbal tea
One scoop of Personal Protein in 4 to 5 oz. of cold water or soy milk

Lunch:
6 oz. of yellowtail snapper in lemon butter
Small mixed salad of lettuce, onions, red peppers, with sprinkled feta
   cheese, garlic dressing
Side of green beans
10 to 12 oz. of club soda, green tea, water, or glass of white wine

Afternoon Snack:
Several rye crisps or wasa bread with goat cheese
10 to 12 oz. of club soda, green tea, or water

Dinner:
8-oz. lean ground beef with Worcestershire sauce
Side of turnips or parsnips with onions
Mixed salad of bibb lettuce, arugula, bamboo shoots, water chestnuts,
   radishes, and scallions, with ginger dressing
10 to 12 oz. of club soda, green tea, water, or glass of red wine

Evening Snack:
One slice of toasted raisin Ezekiel bread with butter, jelly or jam
10 to 12 oz. of club soda, green tea, water, or soy milk

Before Bedtime:
One scoop of Personal Protein in 4 or 5 oz. of cold water

PHYSICALLY INACTIVE PERSON
7-DAY MENU FOR TYPE O

Day 5

Breakfast:

4 oz. of prune juice
Medium bowl of amaranth flakes with banana or blueberries with soymilk
One slice of toasted Essene bread with butter, jelly or jam
Cup of hot parsley or ginger herbal tea
One scoop of Personal Protein in 4 to 5 oz. of water

Lunch:

Grilled or broiled lamb chops with mint jelly
Side of green peas
Side of basmati rice
10 to 12 oz. of club soda, green tea, water, or glass or red wine

Afternoon Snack:

Carob chip cookies with walnuts, or one large apple
10 to 12 oz. of club soda, green tea, or water

Dinner:

Grilled calves liver and onions
Romaine lettuce with dandelion and beet leaves
Two or three artichokes
Side of spinach with leeks
10 to 12 oz. of club soda, green tea, water, or glass of white wine

Evening Snack:

One slice of toasted raisin Ezekiel bread with butter, jelly or jam
10 to 12 oz. of club soda, green tea, water, or soy milk

Before Bedtime:

One scoop of Personal Protein in 4 to 5oz. of cold water

PHYSICALLY INACTIVE PERSON
7-DAY MENU FOR TYPE O

Day 6

Breakfast:
4 oz. of pineapple juice
Medium bowl of cream of rice, cream of kasha, or spelt with currants, blueberries, or elderberries
One slice of Essene bread with butter, jelly or jam
Cup of hot cayenne herbal tea
One scoop of Personal Protein in 4 or 5 oz. of cold water, or soy milk

Lunch:
Cold cucumber soup with onions or leeks
Six ounces albacore tune
Two brown rice cakes
Side of sliced red bell pepper with garlic and olive oil dressing
10 to 12 oz. of club soda, green tea, or water

Afternoon Snack:
6 or 8 figs, or two plums
10 to 12 oz. of club soda, green tea, or water

Dinner:
8 oz. grilled or broiled T-bone steak
Side of collard greens, broccoli and onions, or kale
White rice with aduke or azuki beans with turmeric
10 to 12 oz. of club soda, green tea, water, or glass of red wine

Evening Snack:
Mixed almonds and Macadamia nuts
10 to 12 oz. of club soda, green tea, or water

Before Bedtime:
One scoop of Personal Protein in 4 to 5 oz. of cold water

PHYSICALLY INACTIVE PERSON
7-DAY MENU FOR TYPE O

Day 7

Breakfast:
4 oz. glass of prune juice
Medium bowl of kamut with acceptable fruit and soy milk
One slice of toasted raisin Ezekiel bread with butter, jelly or jam
Cup of hot Chickweed, Fenugreek, or Hops herbal tea
One scoop of Personal Protein in 4 to 5 oz. of cold water

Lunch:
Artichoke pasta with meat sauce, garlic and oil, or white clam sauce
Mixed green salad of romaine lettuce, onions, garlic, okra, asparagus, and
    pinto beans, with miso dressing
10 to 12 oz. of club soda, green tea, water, or glass of white wine

Afternoon Snack:
One large apple or mixed fruits (apricots, figs, prunes, grapes, or dates)
10 to 12 oz. of club soda, green tea, or water

Dinner:
8 oz. of grilled or broiled snapper, rainbow trout, cod, halibut, swordfish,
    or lobster tail
White rice with pinto, or black-eyed peas
Side of escarole, chicory, broccoli or broccoli sprouts, or turnips
10 to 12 oz. of club soda, green tea, water, or glass of white wine

Evening Snack:
Pumpkin seeds and walnuts
10 to 12 oz. of club soda, green tea, or water

Before Bedtime:
One scoop of Personal Protein in 4 to 5 oz. of cold water

Personal Protein available on web site 4blood.com or 1-888-41BLOOD.

Note: Since Os cannot tolerate grains well, and because Essene and Ezekiel bread is highly beneficial with numerous sprouted grains, which don't cause intestinal irritation, they are repeatedly in the diet. Type Os do better than any other type with lean meats and other proteins, so the diet is heavy in protein, supplemented with fruits and vegetables.

PHYSICALLY ACTIVE PERSON
7-DAY MENU FOR TYPE O

Day 1

Breakfast:
Two eggs boiled, poached, or scrambled
3 or 4 slices of turkey bacon
One slice of toasted raisin Ezekiel bread with butter
Cup of hot peppermint herbal tea
Two scoops of Personal Protein in 10 to 12 oz. cold water.

Lunch:
6 oz. of chicken breast
Romaine lettuce with tofu, artichokes, garlic and onions
10 to 12 oz. of club soda, seltzer, water, or green tea

Afternoon Snack:
Protein bar - 20 to 35 grams, or protein shake
10 to 12 oz. club soda, water, or green tea

Dinner:
8 oz. filet mignon in lemon butter
Mixed green salad with red peppers, feta cheese, garlic olive oil dressing
One sweet potato
10 to 12 oz. of club soda, water, green tea, or glass of red wine

Evening Snack:
Pumpkin seeds and walnuts
10 to 12 oz. of club soda, water, green tea, or soy milk

Before Bedtime:
Two scoops of Personal Protein in 10 to 12 oz. cold water

PHYSICALLY ACTIVE PERSON
7-DAY MENU FOR TYPE O

Day 2

Breakfast:
3 or 4 fresh or dried figs
Medium bowl of rice bran or cream of rice
One slice of Essene bread with butter
Cup of hot rosehips herbal tea
Two scoops of Personal Protein in 10 to 12 oz. cold water.

Lunch:
Small can of sockeye salmon with celery, onions, mayonnaise & cayenne
    pepper
Mixed salad of romaine lettuce, broccoli sprouts, leeks, soy beans, and
    parsley
10 to 12 oz. of club soda, water, or green tea

Afternoon Snack:
Protein bar - 20 to 35 grams, or protein shake
10 to 12 oz. of club soda, water, green tea

Dinner:
8 oz. chicken breast in tarragon sauce
Side of spinach
Side of pinto beans with goat cheese and mozzarella
Side of sliced red bell peppers with garlic dill dressing
10 to 12 oz. of club soda, green tea, water, or glass of white wine

Evening Snack:
Mixed pumpkin seeds, walnuts, and Macadamia nuts
10 to 12 oz. of club soda, green tea, or water

Before Bedtime:
Two scoops of Personal Protein in 10 to 12 oz. of cold water

PHYSICALLY ACTIVE PERSON
7-DAY MENU FOR TYPE O

Day 3

Breakfast:
Ground beef with melted soy cheese on toasted Ezekiel bread
Cup hot mulberry herbal tea
Two scoops of Personal Protein in 10 to 12 oz. cold water.

Lunch:
Sliced fresh turkey breast
Mixed green salad with grilled tofu, watercress, endive with garlic olive oil
10 to 12 oz. club soda, green tea, or water

Afternoon Snack:
Protein bar - 20 to 35 grams, or protein shake
10 to 12 oz. of water or green tea

Dinner:
Grilled or broiled 8 oz. flank steak
One medium sweet potato
Side of broccoli or broccoli sprouts
One portobello mushroom with garlic and olive oil
10 to 12 oz. of club soda, green tea, water, or glass of red wine

Evening Snack:
Soy flour bread with tahini (sesame butter)
10 to 12 oz. of club soda, green tea, or water

Before Bedtime:
Two scoops of Personal Protein in 10 to 12 oz. cold water.

PHYSICALLY ACTIVE PERSON
7-DAY MENU FOR TYPE O

Day 4

Breakfast:
4 oz. of apricot juice
Two eggs any style
Three strips of turkey bacon (this is turkey, not pork)
One slice of Essene bread with butter
Cup of hot Sarsaparilla herbal tea
Two scoops of Personal Protein in 10 to 12 oz. cold water.

Lunch:
6 oz. of yellowtail snapper in lemon butter
Mixed salad of lettuce, onions, red peppers, feta cheese, garlic olive oil
Side of green beans
10 to 12 oz. of club soda, green tea, water, or glass of white wine

Afternoon Snack:
Protein bar - 20 to 35 grams, or protein shake
10 to 12 oz. of club soda, water, or green tea

Dinner:
8 oz. lean ground beef with Worcestershire sauce
Side of turnips or parsnips with onions
Side of soy beans, green, brown, or black
10 to 12 oz. of club soda, green tea, water, or glass of red wine

Evening Snack:
One slice of toasted raisin Ezekiel bread with butter
10 to 12 oz. of club soda, green tea, water, or soy milk

Before Bedtime:
Two scoops of Personal Protein in 10 or 12 oz. cold water.
Look for all of these items at your favorite health food store

PHYSICALLY ACTIVE PERSON
7-DAY MENU FOR TYPE O

Day 5

Breakfast:
3 oz. of prune juice
Medium bowl of amaranth flakes with soy milk
One slice of toasted Essene bread with butter
Cup of hot parsley or ginger herbal tea
Two scoops of Personal Protein in 10 to 12 oz. cold water.

Lunch:
Grilled or broiled lamb chops with mint jelly
Side of green peas
Side of kidney beans with melted mozzarella or goat cheese
10 to 12 oz. of club soda, green tea, water, or glass or red wine

Afternoon Snack:
Protein bar - 20 to 35 grams, or protein shake
10 to 12 oz. of club soda, water, green tea

Dinner:
Grilled calves liver and onions
Romaine lettuce with dandelion and beet leaves
Side of soybeans of choice
10 to 12 oz. of club soda, green tea, water, or glass of white wine

Evening Snack:
One slice of toasted Ezekiel bread with butter
10 to 12 oz. of club soda, green tea, water, or soy milk

Before Bedtime:
Two scoops of Personal Protein in 10 to 12 oz. cold water.

PHYSICALLY ACTIVE PERSON
7-DAY MENU FOR TYPE O

Day 6

Breakfast:
Medium bowl of cream of rice, cream of kasha, or spelt
One slice of Essene bread with butter
Cup of hot cayenne herbal tea
Two scoops of Personal Protein in 10 or 12 oz. cold water

Lunch:
Six ounces albacore tune
Two brown rice cakes
Side of sliced red bell pepper, goat cheese with garlic and olive oil dressing
10 to 12 oz. of club soda, green tea, or water

Afternoon Snack:
Protein bar - 20 to 35 grams, or protein shake
10 to 12 oz. of club soda, water, green tea

Dinner:
8 oz. grilled or broiled T-bone steak
Side of collard greens, broccoli and onions, or kale
Aduke or azuki beans with melted mozzarella
10 to 12 oz. of club soda, green tea, water, or glass of red wine

Evening Snack:
Mixed almonds and Macadamia nuts
10 to 12 oz. of club soda, water, green tea

Before Bedtime:
Two scoops of Personal Protein in 10 to 12 oz. of cold water

PHYSICALLY ACTIVE PERSON
7-DAY MENU FOR TYPE O

Day 7

Breakfast:

Medium bowl of kamut with soy milk
One slice of toasted Ezekiel bread with butter
Cup of hot Chickweed, Fenugreek, or Hops herbal tea
Two scoops of Personal Protein in 10 to 12 oz. cold water.

Lunch:

Grilled hamburger with melted mozzarella
Mixed green salad of romaine lettuce, onions, soy beans or tofu, garlic
   olive oil
10 to 12 oz. of club soda, green tea, water, or glass of white wine

Afternoon Snack:

Protein bar - 20 to 35 grams, or protein shake
10 to 12 oz. of club soda, water, green tea

Dinner:

8 oz. of grilled or broiled snapper, rainbow trout, cod, halibut, swordfish,
   or lobster tail
Mixed salad with escarole, chicory, broccoli sprouts, tempeh, and goat
   cheese
10 to 12 oz. of club soda, green tea, water, or glass of white wine

Evening Snack:

Pumpkin seeds, walnuts, and Macadamia nuts
10 to 12 oz. of club soda, water, green tea

Before Bedtime:

Two scoops of Personal Protein in 10 to 12 oz. of cold water

Personal Protein available on web site 4blood.com or 1-888-41BLOOD.

REFERENCES

The following are the references, listed alphabetically, that were relied upon for the writing of this book.

Alfred, JB, "Too much of a good thing? An overemphasis on eating low-fat foods may be contributing to the alarming increase in overweight among US adults," J. Amer Dietetic Assoc. 1995 (4): 417-418.

"American Association of Blood Banks, Technical Manuel, 10th ed." 1990.

Allan, T.M., and Dawson, A.A. "ABO blood groups and ischemic heart disease in men." Brit. Heart J., 30 (1968): 377-82.

Asimov, I., (1959), The Living River. Abelard-Schuman, New York, New York.

Atkins, R., and Herwood, R.W. Dr. Atkin's Diet Revolution, New York: Bantam, 1972.

Atkins, R., Dr. Atkin's New Diet Revolution, New York: M. Evans and Company, 1992.

Bordia, A "Effect of garlic on blood lipids in patients with coronary heart disease," The American Journal of Clinical Nutrition 34(1981), pp. 100-03.

Bodmer, W.F. and Cavalli-Sforza, L.L. (1976). "Genetics, evolution, and Man". Wh.H. Freeman & Co., San Francisco.

Borecci, T.B., et al. "ABO Associations with Blood Pressure, Serum Lipids and Lipoproteins, and Anthroprometric Measures." Human Heredity 1985;5 (3): 161-70.

Boyd, W. C. Genetics and the Races of Man: An Introduction to Modern Physical Anthropology. Boston: Little, Brown, 1950.

Buckwalter, et al. "Ethnologic aspects of the ABO blood groups: Disease associations." JAMA, 1957:327.

Council on Foods and Nutrition "A critique of low-carbohydrate ketogenic weight reduction regimens," JAMA 224(10) 1973, pp 1415-19.

D'Adamo, P.J., et al., "4 Blood Types, 4 Diets, Eat Right For Your Type." G. P. Putnam's Sons, New York, 1996.

Eades, Michael R., Mary Dan, M.D's., "Protein Power," Bantam Books, New York, 1996.

Egger, J. et al. "Is migraine food allergy? A double-blind controlled trial of oligoantigenic diet treatment," Lancet (October 29, 1984, pp. 719-21).

Gittleman, Ann Louise, M.S., Templeton, James, Versace, Candelora "Your Body Knows Best", Simon U Schuster, N.J., 1996.

Green, D., et al., Relationship among Lewis PhenoType, clotting factors, and other Cardiovascular Risk Factors in Young Adults, Department of Medicine, Northwestern University Medical School, Chicago, Il, Journal of Laboratory & Clinical Medicine, (1995).

Garrison, R.J., et al., "ABO Blood Group and Cardiovascular Disease: The Framingham Study." Atherosclerosis 1976 Nov-Dec:25 (2-3):311-8.

Gill, JC., et al., "The Effect of ABO Blood Group on the Diagnosis of Von Willebrand Disease"., Blood 1987 Jun;69 (6) :1691-1695.

Guezennec, Cy., "Role of lipids on endurance capacity in man." Int J Sports Med, 1992; 1992 13(suppl 1):s114-S118.

Harrison, G.A. (ed.) (1977). "Population structure and human variation". Cambridge University Press.

Hickson, JF., and Wolinsky, I., Eds., "Nutrition in Exercise and Sport," 2nd ed., CRC Press 1994; 34,75.

Hirszfeld, L., and Hirszfeld, H. Lancet, 2 (119): 675.

Howells, W.W. (1960). "Mankind in the making: the story of human evolution". Secker and Warburg, London. Penguin, Harmondsworth (1967).

Jia, DX., "Bone Tumor and ABO Blood Type.", Seamen's Hospital, Shanghai. Chung Hua Chung Liu Tsa /chih 1991 May;13 (3):220-222.

Jick, H., Porter, J., "Thrombophlebitis of the Lower Extremities and ABO Blood Type." Arch Intern Med 1978 Oct;138 (10): 1566-1567

Kather, H. et al., "Influences of variation in total energy intake and dietary composition on regulation of fat cell lipolysis in ideal-weight subjects." J. Clin Invest, 1987;80:566-572.

Kramer, FM. Et al., "Long-term follow-up of behavioral treatment for obesity: Patterns of weight gain among men and women." Int J. Obes, 1989;13:123-136.

Kuchi, M., and Jack, A "The Cancer Prevention Diet". New York: St. Martin's, 1983

Kvist, E., et al., "Relationship between Blood Groups and Tumors of the Upper Urinary Tract." Department of Surgery, Sundby Hospital, Copenhagen, Denmark., Scand J. Urol Nephrol 1988;22 (4):289-291.

Manninen, V. "Joint effects of serum triglycerides and LDL cholesterol and HDL cholesterol on coronary heart disease in the Helsinki Heart Study. Implications for treatment." Circulation 85(1) 1992, pp. 365-67.

Marinaccio, M., et al. "Blood Groups of the ABO System and Survival Rate in Gynecologic Tumors." Minerva Ginecol 1995 Mar;47 (3):69-76.

McNeil, W.H., "Plagues and Peoples". New York: Doubleday/ Anchor, 1975.

Meshalkin, E.N., "ABO and Rh blood groups in cardiovascular pathology." Kardiologia 1981 Apr:21 (4): 46-50

Mourant, A.E., Kipec, A.C., & Domaniewska-Sobczak, K. (1978). "Blood groups and diseases". Oxford University Press.

Mourant, A.E., Kopec, A.C., and Domaniewska-Sobczak, K., (1978). The genetics of the Jews. Clarendon Press, Oxford.

Muller, W.A. et al. "The influence of the antecedent diet upon glucagon and insulin secretion," New England Journal of Medicine 285(86) (1971), pp. 1450-4.

Muschel, L. "Blood groups, disease and selection." Bacteriological Rev., 30,2 (1966):427-41.

Neumann, JK. et al., "Relationship between Blood Groups and Behavior Patterns in Men who have had Myocardial Infarction.", James H. Quillen College of Medicine, East Tennessee State University, Johnson City, TN., South Med J. 1991 Feb;84 (2): 214-218.

Nachbar, M.S., et al. "Lectins in the U.S. diet: A survey of lectins in commonly consumed foods and a review of the literature." Amer. J. Clin. Nut., 33 (1980): 233845.

Next Nutrition Special Report, The IsoCaloric "No Diet" Fat Burning Handbook, (1996).

Nomi, T., and Besher, A. You are Your Blood Type. New York: Pocket, 1983.

Phillips, B., (1997), Sports Supplement Review (3rd Ed.),

Pritikin, N., and McGrady, P. The Pritikin Program for Diet and Exercise. New York: Grosset & Dunlap. 1979.

Race, R.R., and Sanger, R. Blood Groups in Man. Oxford, England: Blackwell Scientific, 1975.

Reaven, G.M., et al. "Hypertension as a Disease of Carbohydrate and Lipoprotein Metabolism," The American Journal of Medicine 87 (suppl. 6A) 1989, pp. 6a-2S-6A-6S.

Reaven, G.M., and Hollenbeck, C., "Variation of insulin stimulation glucose uptake in healthy individuals with normal glucose tolerance." J Clin Endocrinol Metab, 1987;64:1169-1173.

Rickman, F. et al. "Changes in serum cholesterol during the Stillman diet." JAMA 228(1974, p. 54).

Roberts, J.A. Fraser and Pembrey, M.E. (1985). An introduction to medical genetics (8th Ed.) Oxford University Press.

Rihmer, Z, Arato M., "ABO Blood Groups in Manic-Depressive Patients.", J Affect Discord 1981 Mar;3 (1):1-7.

Saynor, R. "Effects of omega-3 fatty acids on serum lipids," Lancet2 (1984 pp.696-7).

Schmid, R., Traditional Foods Are your Best Medicine. New York: Ballantine, 1987

Sears, B., "Enter the Zone", Regan Books, 1995.

Seaton, TB, et al., "Thermic effect of medium-chain and long chain triglycerides in man." Am Clin Nutr, 1986;44:630-634.

Simopoulos, A., "Omega-3 fatty acids in health and disease and in growth and development." Am J Clin Nutr, 1991;54:438-463.

Stern, C. (1973). "Principles of human genetics (3rd Ed.)". W.H. Freeman & C., San Francisco

Swislocki, AM, et al., "Insulin suppression of plasma free fatty acid concentration in normal individuals or patients with Type II (NIDDM) diabetes." 1987;30:622.

Takeuchi, H., et al., "Diet-induced thermogenesis is lower in rats fed a lard diet than those fed a high oleic acid safflower oil diet, a safflower oil diet or a linseed oil diet.", J Nutr, 1995;125920-925.

Tills, D., Kopec, A.C., and Tills, R.E. (1983), The distribution of the human blood groups: Supplement 1. Oxford University Press.

Tushchenko, G.H., et al., "Blood Groups ABO, MN and Rh in Diseases of the Cardiovascular System"Genetika 1975:11(1) :155-7

Vioque, J., Walker, AM, "Pancreatic Cancer and ABO Blood Types: A study of Cases and Controls." Med Clin (Barc) 1991 May 25;96 (20):761-764.

Wasserman, DH., et al., "Interaction of gut and liver in nitrogen metabolism during exercise." Metab, 1991;40:307-314.

Wintrobe, M. M, (1980), Blood, Pure and Eloquent, A Story of Discovery, of People, and of Ideas., McGraw-Hill Book Company, San Francisco.

Wong, F., et al, "Longitudinal Study of the Association Between ABO blood phenoType and total serum cholesterol (TC) Level as Examined in the Japanese Population." Genetic Epidemiology 1992:9 (6):405-18.

Yamashita, S., and Melmed, S., "Effects of insulin on rat anterior pituitary cells: Inhibition of growth hormone secretion and MRNA levels." Diabetes, 1986;35:440-447.

The following partial research subjects are an indication of the ages and diseases that our research has shown each blood type lives to and dies from.

TYPE A RESEARCH SUBJECTS

LEGEND: ()* =STILL ALIVE

Leon F., extensive heart disease, 1st heart attack 52, hypertension from 22, smoker, fatal heart attack 59.

Mitchell F., extensive heart disease, 1st heart attack 47, smoker, fatal heart attack 50.

Leonard F., mild diabetes, no signs of heart disease, fatal heart attack 71. Longest life in fathers family.

Mary F., high blood pressure 21, blind 26, fatal heart attack 32.

Max F., high blood pressure, diabetes, smoked, drank, fatal heart attack 64.

Etta K., no warning, appeared in good health, fatal heart attack 68.

Max K., hypertension, extensive heart disease, smoker, gambler, fatal heart attack 65.

William S., extensive heart disease, diabetes, fatal heart attack 64.

Robert E., no known diseases, 1st heart attack 62, fatal heart attack 66.

Nancy C., Ellison-Zollinger disease, stomach tumor, smoker, drinker, arthritis, (64)*.

Frank W., deudonal ulcer, cancer-kidney, cancer-prostate, (84)* Oldest ever in his family, and in research.

Lorraine L., vegetarian, no medical problems, (66)*.

Lorraine's Father (Pearl), heart attack 57.

Lorraine's Mother (Pearl), heart attack 73.

Jack H., died of prostate cancer 65.

Edward S., heart attack 53, heart failure and death 61.

Irwin C., very active, sudden heart attack 69.

Sam R., smoker, high blood pressure, died of cancer of liver 67.

Shirley S., high blood pressure, diabetes, died complications of diabetes 65.

Melvin S., diabetes, high blood pressure, died of heart attack 67.

Roger W., died of stomach cancer 54.

On Line, Male, died of heart attack 54.

Judy H., gallbladder removed 18, ITP Idiopathic Thrombo Cyto Penic Pupia 29, now (54)*.

William W., died of heart disease 61.

Nelly B., died of cancer of liver 40.

Robert T., died of heart attack 52.

Emmy H., high blood pressure, hypertension, age (63)*.

Philip F., high blood pressure, overweight, age (38)*.

John F., heart valve problems, high blood pressure, age (65)*.

Maritza F., high blood pressure, age (63)*.

Sylvester A., died suddenly heart attack 65.

Michele D., died of cancer 41.

Andy A., anemia, age (29)*.

William A., heart disease, bypass surgery, age (65)*.

Floyd F., high blood pressure, age (49)*.

John F., died heart disease 60.

Anolia S., low blood pressure, vegetarian, age (51)*.

Lawrence N., diabetes, looks older than age (55)*.

George N., health and fitness nut, died of cancer 82.

Larry L., died of cancer 50.

John G., died of pancreatic cancer 73.

Henry B., died of cancer 58.

Albert K., died of heart attack 43.

David T., died of cancer 65.

Jala D., died of heart attack 63.

Frank M., died of cancer 64.

Mark C, died of stomach cancer 53.

Robert W., died of cancer 65.

Sandy M., diabetes, high blood pressure, thyroid problems, age (63)*.

Robert K., extensive heart disease, bypass surgery, died 63.

Stanley H., died of cancer 70.

Leroy O., died of heart failure 68.

Frankie, O, died of cancer 57.

Lily G., breast cancer, hip & knee replacement, arthritis, age (62)*.

Robert B., died suddenly heart attack 37.

Carson S., died of cancer 62.

Abraham P., suddenly of cardiac arrest 68.

Pedro V., died of heart attack 55.

Carol B., diagetes, high blood pressure, heart attack, age (69)*.

Billy X., high blood pressure, angina, age (69)*.

Robert X., died of heart attack 56.

William R., high blood pressure, died of cancer 61.

Manuel G., fatty mass on liver, memory problems, previously very active physical work, age (62)*.

George G., high blood pressure, panic attacks, bi-polar illness, kidney stones, age (43)*.

Willomena P., seizures since birth, age (17)*.

Shirley R., spastic colon, irritable bowel syndrome, age (40)*.

Elizabeth R., cervical cancer, died of massive heart attack 58.

John R., died of cancer 66.

Arthur S., high blood pressure, age (59)*.

Joe G., high blood pressure, otherwise good health, age (79)*.

Ruth R., minor eye problem, otherwise good health, age (78)*.

David G., died of a heart attack, age 69.

Edward W., died of lung cancer, age 56.

Hannah W., died of cancer of the stomach, age 42.

Victor P., died of sudden heart attack, age 35.

Marion F., died of cancer of the liver, age 72.

Jose V., died of heart disease, age 70.

Joel L., died of cancer, age 50.

Jose P., died of cancer, age 61.

Robert S., died of cancer, age 54.

Robert S., died of a sudden heart attack, age 46.

Catherine S., died of lung cancer, age 70.

Lillian S., died of cancer of the pancreas, age 49.

Joseph H., died of cancer, age 65.

Rene G., died from complications from diabetes and heart disease, age 55.

Charles K., died of a heart attack, age 57.

Eleanor C., died of heart disease, age 77.

Pilar M., died of a heart attack, age 57.

Henry H., died of non-Hodgkins lymphoma, age 63.

Fang Y., died from undisclosed illness, age 81.

Lazaro R., no medical problems, age (40)*.

Maria R., suffers from arthritis, age (64)*

Roberto R., has no medical problems, age (68)*.

Joseph V., died of cancer, age 64.

Manuel P., died of cancer of the prostate, age 63.

Emelio F., died of complications of diabetes, age 71.

Gustavo R., died of heart attack, age 66.

Estelle M., died of cancer of the cervix, age 37.

Bernard F., died of cancer, age 64.

TYPE B RESEARCH SUBJECTS

LEGEND: ( )* =STILL ALIVE

Anita F., spastic colon, irritable bowel syndrome, psoriasis, cancer of colon, angioplasty, age (73)*.

Sophie M., diverticulitis, hip replacement, age (84)*.

Shirley G., brain tumor, bi-polar illness, kidney removed, age (78)*.

Fannie K., bi-polar illness, high blood pressure, enlarged heart, died heart failure 78.

Morris K., mild diabetes, double hernia, died suddenly after insulin shot, age 78.

Harold M., extremely healthy until diagnosis malignant melanoma, died 2 years later, age 81.

John M., undiagnosed illness, extremely allergic to peanuts, chronic fatigue syndrome, age (54)*.

Susan G., spinal disorder, multiple undiagnosed illnesses, age (53)*.

Morjorie G., excellent health, age (53)*.

Bruce G., excellent health, age (55)*.

Gary K., polio as child, carries a limp, general good health, age (50)*.

Herb W., polio as child, 1 diminished leg, high blood pressure, diabetes, drinks, smokes, age (64)*.

William K., died of prostate cancer 75.

Gloria K., heart attack 67, mostly recovered at age (74)*.

Rona R., Lupus age 24, unknown outcome.

Gloria C., enlarged heart, smoked, died complications of emphysema 92.

David S., 1st heart attack 42, 2nd heart attack 45, smokes, drinks, shows no heart damage, no medications.

Rose B., no heart disease, slight arthritis, age (90)*.

William B., died of heart attack 72.

Estelle G., smokes, mild heart attack 72, blockage corotid arteries, age (72)*.

Katherine W., diabetes, high blood pressure, gout, undiagnosed illnesses, age (56)*.

Walter W., excellent health 42.

Shirley T., high blood pressure, high cholesterol, age (70)*.

Woodrow C., mild diabetes, no medication, age (61)*.

Maria A., excellent health (74)*.

Irving B., heart disease, bypass surgery, age (71)*.

Ruth E., excellent health, age (74)*.

Robert G., died of natural causes 84.

Armad D., died from complications of emphysema 79.

Mary G., died of cancer 74.

Howard M., Parkinsons disease age (64)*.

Charles K., died of Lupus, age 64.

Nayland C., diabetes, smokes, high cholesterol, 900 triglycerides, age (63)*.

Sol G., excellent health, age (73)*.

Richard S., died of pulmonary disease 73.

Florence F., died of natural causes 87.

June G., high blood pressure, otherwise good health, age (78)*.

Arthur L., hip replacement, shoulder surgery, almost died from infection after surgery, age (71)*.

Mortimer E., died from a lengthy bout with cancer, age 83.

Carlis J., numerous cancers throughout body, brain tumor, given up for dead many times, age (78)*.

Lucile W., died of a heart attack, age 80.

Bernard S., died of complications from diabetes, age 81.

Edgar H., died of multiple myeloma, age 65.

Lillian N., died of natural causes, age 85.

Millie F., lupus & multiple sclerosis since age 25, now (34)*.

Mitch B., no medical problems, age (40)*.

Bernard B., hip replacement otherwise healthy, age (62)*.

Lillian B., no medical problems, age (62)*.

Isadore L., died of natural causes, age 88.

Myrtle B., died of heart disease, age 81.

Wilbur W., died of natural causes, age 84.

Hy A., died after a long illness, age 76.

Herman P., died of natural causes, age 95.

Jerome W., died after a prolonged illness, age 62.

Hyman G., died of natural causes, age 90.

Alan B., died of respiratory failure, age 79.

Luther S., died of natural causes, age 92.

Bernard F., died of natural causes, age 84.

Helen N., died of cancer, age 84.

Sally R., died of Parkinson's Disease and Alzheimers Disease, age 96.

Jean J., died of cancer, age 67.

Vertner H., has no medical problems, age (55)*.

Miriam N., died of natural causes, age 85.

Betty R., died of pneumonia, age 89.

Isadore B., had ulcer, but no longer, good health, age (79)*.

Esther S., died of natural causes, age 95.

Helen M., died of natural causes, age 92.

Dorothy W., died of heart disease, age 89.

Evelyn T., died of pneumonia, age 88.

John B., died of cancer, age 82.

Ellen R., died of Lupus, age 39.

Brigit P., died of multiple sclerosis, age 51.

Louis S., died of Lou Gherig's disease, age 49.

Margaret S., died of cerebral palsy, age 86.

Ivan V., is in excellent health, age (38)*.

Abraham E., died of complications of pneumonia, age 83.

Charlie S., died of natural causes, age 78.

Juan P., died of a brain tumor, age 69.

Rafael I., died of lung cancer, age 78.

Ruth N., (Israeli), excellent health, age (32)*.

Miguel R., Sr., no medical problems, age (70)*.

Shirley L., suffers from high blood pressure, arthritis, age (91)*.

Phyllis C., suffers from arthritis, age (76)*.

Bernard C., no health problems, drinks heavily, smokes, age (64)*.

Henry G., professor/researcher, still working, age (91)*.

Sidney W., died of heart failure, age 76.

Paula W., died of natural causes, age 89.

Precilla S., died of multiple sclerosis, age 78.

Isaac F., died of natural causes, age 92.

Maria G., is in good health, age (32)*.

Fara G., suffers from lupus, age (59)*.

Morris K., died of pneumonia, age 86.

Pearl K., died of old age, age 91.

Seymour R., died of multiple scleroses, age 69.

Richard K., suffers from neuro Fibro myalgia, age (48)*.

Harold R., died from a series of strokes, age 81.

TYPE AB RESEARCH SUBJECTS

LEGEND: ( )* =STILL ALIVE

Gene F., died of cancer 74.

Terry S., hypertension, high blood pressure, age (42)*.

Cathryn L., Platelet Aggregation Disorder, age (49)*.

Ed B., gallbladder removed, otherwise good health, age (65)*.

Judith B., excellent health, age (61)*.

Jens K., excellent health, age (26)*.

Perry A., malignant melanoma on back 36, age (38)*.

David S., excellent health, age (57)*.

Safta D., excellent health, age (57)*.

Livingston C., died from bleeding ulcers 47.

Susan S., Fibro Cystic Ovaries, anemic, clotting, cramping menstrual cycles, age (49)*.

Allen K., extreme arthritis, 2 hip replacements, 1 knee replacement, age (68)*.

Gale R., tubes tied 27, irregular, clotting, cramping, menstrual cycles, age (35)*.

Roberta S., diabetes, angina, age (41)*.

Abraham S., no medical problems, age (78)*. Oldest AB known in research.

Anna G., excellent health, age (44)*.

William W., rapid heart beat, takes beta blockers, gout, arthritis, age (70)*.

Lauren M., migraine headaches, anemia, profuse, irregular, frequent, clotting menstrual cycles, age (38)*.

Samuel S., died of natural causes, age 88.

Joan K., died of Parkinson's disease, age 67.

Mario R., died of natural causes, age 73.

Janet L., died of natural causes, age 89.

Richard B., suffers from high blood pressure, age (51)*.

Wayne S., suffers from high blood pressure, age (67)*.

Arthur R., has no major health problems, age (62)*.

Beatrice M., suffers from irregular menstrual cycles, excess bleeding, clotting, age (44)*.

Bruce T., is in excellent health, tried body building but can't build muscle, runs a lot, age (38)*.

Ari B., died of congestive heart failure, age 53.

Jennie R., died of breast cancer, age 70.

Beatrice C., died of a massive stroke, age 79.

Moshe N., (Israeli), excellent health, very difficult to build muscle by working out, age (33)*

Jeffrey F., bi-polar illness, age (51)*.

Miguel R., Jr., 1st black met that is AB, overweight, trouble building muscle, age (32)*.

Asa M., suffered diabetes prior to regular exercise program, age (73)*.

Frank L., suffered previous HBP, weight training 4 x week, trouble building muscle, look great, age (70)*.

Dean S., overweight, eats everything, no health problems, age (60)*.

Mike C., lost leg in accident, otherwise excellent health, age (38)*.

Mary Ann C., AB-, 5 miscarriages, very sensitive to food, smokes, drinks but general good health, age (59)*.

Roland P., in good health, age (56)*.

Allan L., died of melanoma, age 48.

Arthur S., is in good health, age (66)*.

Rosalie B., suffers from irregular menstrual cycles, clotting, bleeding, age (41)*.

Bert R., died of heart disease, age 69.

Marie F., is in excellent health, age (67)*.

Adelaide M., died of a heart attack, age 73.

William C., died of cancer of the prostate, age 68.

Sanford D., died of cancer, age 58.

Archibald P., died of heart failure, age 73.

Denise A., died of breast cancer, age 49.

Arnold M., died of a sudden heart attack, age 74.

Willem F., died of prostate cancer, age 59.

Franklin R., died of pneumonia, age 70.

Bernard P., died of complications of diabetes, age 68.

Patrick D., died of malignant melanoma, age 43.

Anita S., died of cancer of the cervix, age 44.

David H., died of heart disease, age 71.

Arnold M., suffers from high blood pressure, age (47)*.

Stephen B., died of congestive heart failure, age 66.

Mario A., died of cancer of the prostate, age 71.

Elio P., died of a sudden heart attack, age 53.

Susan R., died of breast cancer, age 44,

Cynthia P., died of uterine cancer, age 48.

Bradley M., is in excellent health, age (74)*.

Mei T., has irregular menstrual cycles, profuse bleeding and clotting, age (31)*.

Arthur C., died of a sudden heart attack, age 67.

Beatrice R., died of complications of diabetes, age 69.

Osvaldo N., died of malignant melanoma, age 62.

Katherine D., died of lupus, age 55.

William D., has severe arthritis, high blood pressure, age (65)*.

Sylvester M., died of emphysema, age 67.

Barry S., died of cardiac arrest, age 73.

Ruth H., died of congestive heart failure, age 69.

Mitchell L., died of a sudden heart attack, age 41.

Paul M., died of cancer, age 66.

John D., died of heart failure after a series of heart attacks, age 68.

Louis F., had a hip replacement, otherwise in good health, age (73)*.

Henry V., suffers from heart disease, high blood pressure, age (73)*.

George A., died of cancer of the pancreas, age 69.

Barbara C., died of heart disease, age 79.

Frederick M., died of a brain tumor, age 62.

Peter R., died of cancer, age 70.

Armando A., died of a heart attack, age 65.

Luis K., died of congestive heart failure, age 76.

Frank P., died of leukemia, age 63.

Shirley O., died of a heart attack, age 73.

Nadia H., has severe arthritis, age (77)*.

James R., died of cancer of the liver, age 60.

Mary P., died of breast cancer, age 49.

Cary G., has heart disease, high blood pressure, age (72)*.

Javier B., is in excellent health, age 64.

Mary N., has mild arthritis, otherwise in excellent health, age (72)*.

Robert K., suffers from bi-polar illness, high blood pressure, age (47)*.

Carol G., died of lung cancer, age 76.

Kathy Y., died of cancer of the thyroid, age 68.

Stanley E., is in excellent health, age (73)*.

Sidney B., has high blood pressure and cancer of the kidney, age (75)*.

Louise M., died of cancer of the stomach, age 61.

Lisa L., has double irregular menstrual periods, clotting, cramping, Crohn's Disease, age (40)*.

Randy J., has no medical problems, age (32)*.

Cynthia A., died of a heart attack, age 59.

Jack O., died of cancer of the prostate, age 63.

TYPE O RESEARCH SUBJECTS

LEGEND: ()* =STILL ALIVE

Jack M., excellent health, mild arthritis, age (77)*.

Harold P., mild arthritis, died from sudden stroke age 91.

George D., emphysema, arthritis, triple bypass, smoker, high blood pressure, age (80)*.

Mario E., died from stroke 90.

John P., ulcers, arthritis, high blood pressure, heart attack 76, died of heart failure 91.

Juana A., died of heart failure 100.

Aurelio P., mild arthritis, age (78)*.

Rene R., excellent health, age (70)*.

Robert L., heart disease, quad bypass 47, 4 stints 65, burst aorta and heart attack 66, coma 4 weeks, cancer removed from face 67, double hernia, heart surgery 68, recovering well, age (68)*.

Florence V., Alzheimers disease, died in sleep 87.

Spike V., eight (8) heart attacks, two (2) strokes. 1st heart attack 54, 8th heart attack 76, died stroke 78.

Rose H., high blood pressure, 2 malignant cysts age 89 & 90, excellent health (91)*.

Max H., borderline diabetes, died from series of strokes 88.

Fannie K., healthy entire life, died from stroke 93.

Issac K., died from undiagnosed cause 99.

Michael H., heart attack 65, no blockages, no damage, age (66)*.

William B., died of lung failure 100.

Cecile P., died of heart failure 96.

George K., smoker, drinker, arthritis, 1st stroke 84, died of 2nd stroke 87.

Evelyn G., drinker, smoker, ulcers, diabetes, severe arthritis, died of stroke 89.

Susie N., died in her sleep, age 90.

Kenneth M., died from complications of stroke, age 91.

Irving K., heart attack 43, high blood pressure, doing well, age (47)*.

Katherine L., mild arthritis, died from stroke, age 86.

Stephen S., 1st stroke 61, died from 2nd stroke 72.

Gil J., diabetes, two (2) heart attacks, numerous strokes (more than 10) smoker, alive at (77)*.

Ethel O., mild arthritis, otherwise excellent health, age (80)*.

Jose L., smokes heavily, tortured in Nicaraguan prison, age (67)*.

Maria L., excellent health, age (94)*.

Binicio L., died of natural causes, age 88.

Ben H., colon cancer, Alzheimers disease, chain smoker, died age 84.

Clarence K., emphysema, numerous strokes leading to his death, age 85.

Willomet P., excellent health, age 68.

Mercedes H., high blood pressure, otherwise healthy, age (49)*.

Sara H., excellent health, age (65)*.

Pedro H., excellent health, age (59)*.

William M., excellent health, age (70)*.

Cherie M., excellent health, age (46)*.

Linda T., mild arthritis, high cholesterol, high blood pressure, age (89)*.

Walter C., excellent health, age (63)*.

Kathrine S., died of old age 98.

John S., died of old age, age 97.

Mary F., excellent health, age (37)*.

William F., excellent health, age (63)*.

Sylvia C., excellent health, age (60)*.

Angel G., excellent health, age (37)*.

Linda N., excellent health, age (54)*.

Herbert H., emphysema, died of natural causes 85.

Julia H., mild arthritis, age (78)*.

Alan H., excellent health, age (50)*.

Carmen G., died of natural causes, age 104.

Edna H., died of natural causes, age 100.

Bernard M., died of natural causes, age 92.

May B., died of natural causes, age 97.

Martin L., died of natural causes, age 88.

Burgess M., Alzheimers disease, death from malignant melanoma. age 89.

John B., died of natural causes, age 99.

Gretta F., died of heart failure, age 92.

Billie G., died from complications of diabetes, age 101.

Samuel J., suffered blood disorder, died of old age and neglect, age 103.

Ralph C., cancer of throat, tongue, cheek, age 51, smoker, drinker, today cancer free, age (65)*.

John S., hepatitis, otherwise excellent health, age (50)*.

Caryl S., died of inflammation of colon after eating walnuts, age 86.

Helen S., perontonitis, other healthy, age (86)*.

Louise L., died from complications of Alzheimers, age 87.

Sayde K., died of natural causes, age 99.

Morris K., died after a series of strokes, age 78.

Victor B., excellent health, age (57)*.

Richard P., excellent health, age (58)*.

Linda P., had gallbladder removed, otherwise excellent health, age (56)*.

Harold B., excellent health, age (64)*.

Charles B., lost left hand 24, lost kidney, 71, excellent health, age (90)*.

Donald B., excellent health, age (66)*.

Eugene B., excellent health, age (64)*.

Joyce B., severe arthritis, irregular heartbeat, otherwise healthy, age (63)*.

Karen W., high blood pressure, age (61)*.

Linda W., high blood pressure, emphysema, age (83)*.

Mary O., died of natural causes, age 104.

Rene R., excellent health, age (71)*.

Sol C., aortic aneuyism, mild arthritis, high blood pressure, age (87)*.

Al G., excellent health, age (74)*.

Kathy C., slight irregular heartbeat, otherwise excellent health, age (43)*.

Richard C., excellent health, age (66)*.

Roberta C., arthritis, heart disease, functional GI problems, diverticulitis, hardening of arteries, age (96)*.

John C., heart attack 57, age (63)*.

Linda C., exzema, otherwise healthy, age (58)*.

Sahara G., high blood pressure, slight arthritis, age (73)*.

Vieginio C., stroke in 50's, fully recovered, died from stroke, age 87.

Rosario P., died of colon cancer, age 83.

Elouise P., died of natural causes, age 90.

Harold R., died of old age 92.

Annie R., died of natural causes, age 91.

Ollie D., died of natural causes, age 96.

Shirley P., heart condition (MVP) age 40, died lung cancer after heart attack, age 67.

Steve A., ankylosing spondolitis, ulcers, heart attack 40, gastritis, colitis, age (41)*.

John A., ankylosing spondolitis, otherwise healthy, age (51)*.

Wesley G., died of heart failure, age 86.

Jabin W., died of old age, age 90.

Harold G., died of heart failure, age 94.

John D., died of complications of diabetes, age 81.

Jerome G., died of heart failure, age 89.

Harvey M., died of cancer of the prostate, age 64.

Georgiana B., died of natural causes, age 92.

Bessie S., had severe arthritis, died of natural causes, age 93

Amino Acids: These are nitrogen containing, carbon-based, organic compounds that serve as the building blocks from which protein (and muscle) are made.

Anabolic: Anabolism is the actual building process of tissues, mainly muscle. It occurs by taking substances from the blood essential for growth and repair and using them to stimulate reactions, which produce tissue synthesis.

Antioxidants: These are nutrients that minimize tissue oxidation and help control free radicals and their harmful effects.

BCAAs: Branch Chain Amino Acids. Amino acids are namely: leucine, isoleucine and valine.

Biological Value (BV): This is the measure of protein quality, assessed by how well a given food or food mixture supports nitrogen retention in humans.

Carbohydrates: Organic compounds containing carbon, hydrogen and oxygen. They are a very effective fuel source for the body. The different types of carbohydrates include starches, sugars, and fibers. Carbohydrates contain four calories per gram and are classified into three groups – monosaccharides, disaccharides, and polysaccharides. Glucose – blood sugar – is a carbohydrate used by every cell in the body as fuel.

Catabolic: Opposite of anabolic. It means the breakdown of tissue. Catabolic states occur with disease, infection, injury, intense training, strict dieting, and immobilization. Catabolic conditions are not conducive to lean muscle mass gains; in fact, they typically cause a loss of lean muscle mass.

Cholesterol: This is a Type of lipid (fat) which, although most widely know as a "bad fat", implicated in promoting heart disease and stroke, is a vital component in the production of many steroid hormones in the body. It also plays a vital role in proper cell-membrane structure and functioning. It's the substrate for bile-acid synthesis, as well as sex hormone and Vitamin D. synthesis. There are different types of cholesterol: namely, HDL (good form), and LDL (bad form).

Cortisol: This is one of the primary catabolic hormones in the body. However, catabolism, or the breakdown of body tissue, is not the only function of cortisol. It is typically secreted in response to physical trauma or prolonged stress. Its functions include controlling inflammation, increasing muscular catabolism and glycolysis (the energy yielding conversion of glucose to lactic acid), suppressing immune response, and maintaining normal vascular circulation and renal function, among others. Suppressing cortisol production at times during the day may help bodybuilders avoid excess muscle breakdown. Cortisol is essential for survival.

EAAs: Essential Amino Acids, which are necessary and vital to life, indispensable to body function, and are made up of the following: Leucine, Isoleucine, Valine, Lysine, Threonine, Methionne, Phenylalanine, and Tryptophan.

Enzyme: This is a protein molecule that acts as a "helper" in thousands of chemical reactions in the body, including: digestion of food, hormone production, muscle cell repair, and literally thousands of other bodily functions.

Fat: This is one of the macronutrients. Fat contains nine calories per gram; it has the most calories of all the macronutrients. Dietary fats may also be referred to as lipids or triglycerides. Fats act as structural components for all cell membranes and supply necessary chemical substrates for hormone production. There are two types of fats-saturated "bad" fat and unsaturated "good" fat.

Saturated Fat: This is "bad" fat. It is called "saturated" because it contains no open spots on its "carbon skeletons." Saturated fats include myristic acid, palmitic acid, stearic acid, arachidic acid, and lignoceric acid. These bad fats have been shown to raise cholesterol levels in the body. Sources of these fats include animal foods and hydrogenated vegetable oils, such as margarine. These fats serve no biological function in the body, other than to supply calories and wreak havoc in our arteries.

Unsaturated Fat: This is "good" fat. It is called "unsaturated" because it has one or more open "carbon spots." Unsaturated fats can be divided into two categories: polyunsaturated and monounsaturated. Unsaturated fats have been shown to help reduce cholesterol and triglyceride levels in the blood. This category of fats includes the essential fatty acids linoleic and linolenic. The main sources of these fats are plant foods.

Free Radicals: Highly reactive molecules possessing unpaired electrons produced during metabolism of food and energy production. Free radicals are believed to contribute to the molecular damage and death of vital body cells. They may be a factor in aging or disease and may ultimately contribute to death. Antioxidants help neutralize free radicals.

Essential Fatty Acids: These are fats that our bodies can't make, so we must obtain them through our diets. These fats (which include linoleic and linolenic acid) are very important to hormone production, as well as cellular synthesis and integrity. Flaxseed oil is a good source of these acids.

Glucose: This is the simplest sugar molecule. It's also the main sugar found in blood and is used as a basic fuel for the body. When you eat complex carbohydrates, the body breaks them down into glucose. Glucose is also found in various fruits, but not in as high concentrations as sucrose and fructose, two other sugars. However, when you eat too much glucose, it's converted to fatty acids and triglycerides by the liver and fatty tissue.

Glycemic Index: An index based upon how quickly insulin enters the bloodstream after certain foods are eaten.

HDL: This stands for "high-density lipoprotein." It is one of the sub-categories of cholesterol, typically thought of as the "good" cholesterol. HDL cholesterol is the form typically used to clear fats from the system, therefore not lending itself to the formation of plaque in your arteries that can cause heart attacks. You may be able to raise your HDL cholesterol levels by ingesting quality unsaturated fats like flaxseed oil, or drinking a glass of red wine on a daily basis. Exercise has also been shown to increase HDL levels.

LDL: This stands for "low-density lipoprotein" and is a sub-category of cholesterol typically thought of as the "bad" cholesterol. LDL is the type of cholesterol that circulates throughout the bloodstream, sometimes leading to heart disease. Levels of LDL cholesterol can be elevated by ingestion of saturated fats and lack of exercise.

Glycogen: This is the principal storage form of carbohydrate energy (glucose) which is reserved in muscles and in the liver. Muscles full of glycogen look and feel full/pumped.

Glucagon: This is a hormone responsible for helping maintain proper sugar levels. When blood sugar levels go too low, glucagon activates glucose production in the liver, as well as regulates the release of glycogen from muscle cells. Eventually it may cause the catabolism of muscle cell proteins for glucose. This is considered a catabolic hormone.

Hypoglycemia: This is low blood sugar/glucose levels, resulting in anxiety, fatigue, perspiration, delirium, and in severe cases, coma. Hypoglycemia occurs most commonly in diabetics where it is due to either insulin overdose or inadequate intake or carbohydrates. Temporary hypoglycemia is common in athletes and can be overcome with the ingestion of carbohydrates.

Insulin: This is an anabolic hormone secreted by the pancreas that aids the body in maintaining proper blood sugar levels and promoting glycogen storage. Insulin secretion speeds the movement of nutrients through the bloodstream and into muscle for growth. When chronically elevated, as with a high-carbohydrate diet, insulin can cause you to gain fat.

Ketones: These are organic chemical compounds resulting from the breakdown of triglycerides. They are used as an energy source in the body during very low carbohydrate diets.

Lectin: Proteins with agglutinating (glue or clotting) properties that may affect your blood in positive or negative ways. Dangerous lectins target different organs and body systems causing damage to the area to which they attach.

Linoleic Acid: This is an essential fatty acid and, more specifically, an omega-6 polyunsaturated fatty acid. Good sources of this fatty acid are safflower and soybean oils.

Linolenic Acid: This is an essential fatty acid and, more precisely, an omega-3 polyunsaturated fatty acid. It is found in high concentrations in flaxseed oil.

Lipid: This is simply another name for dietary fats or triglycerides.

Metabolism: The utilization of nutrients by the body for both anabolic and catabolic processes. It is the process by which substances come into the body and the rate at which they are utilized.

Minerals: Naturally occurring inorganic substances that are essential for human life and play a role in many vital metabolic processes.

Nitrogen: This is an element that distinguishes proteins from other substances and allows them to form various structural units in our bodies, including enzymes and muscle cells.

Nitrogen Balance: This is when the daily intake of nitrogen from proteins equals the daily excretion of nitrogen. A negative nitrogen balance occurs when the excretion of nitrogen exceeds the daily intake and is often seen when muscle is being lost. A positive nitrogen balance is often associated with muscle growth.

Nutrients: These are components of food that help nourish the body; that is, they provide energy or serve as "building materials." Nutrients include carbohydrates, fats, proteins, vitamins, minerals, water, etc.

Oxidation: This is the process of cellular decomposition and breakdown. Oxidation produces free radicals.

Proteins: Highly complex nitrogen-containing compounds found in all animal and vegetable tissues. They are made up of amino acids and are essential for growth and repair in the body. A gram of protein contains four calories. Those from animal sources are high in biological value since they contain the essential amino acids. Those from vegetable sources contain some but not all of the essential amino acids. Proteins are broken down by the body to produce amino acids, which are used to build new proteins. Proteins are the building blocks of muscle, enzymes, and some hormones.

Complete Proteins: These are proteins, which contain all the essential amino acids in the right balance.

Incomplete Proteins: These are proteins that lack or are low in one or more of the essential amino acids.

Triglyceride: This is the scientific name for a common dietary fat. The backbone of the molecule is a glycerol molecule, which is connected to three fatty acid molecules. Triglycerides are also called fats or lipids.

Vitamins: These are organic compounds which are vital to life, indispensable to bodily function, and needed in minute amounts. They are non-caloric, essential nutrients. Many of them function as coenzymes, supporting a multitude of biological functions.

FOODS	GLYCEMIC INDEX

White Rice, Puffed Rice, Rice Cakes, Rice Pasta
Rice Chex
Puffed Wheat
Wheat Bread-gluten free
French Baguette
Fava Beans
Parsnips
Pretzels
Maltose & Glucose

110+^

Breakfast Cereals in General
Whole Wheat Bread, White Bread
Crackers, Cookies
Carrots, Beets, Pumpkin, Watermelon
Baked, Mashed, Fried Potato
Snack Food and Confectionery

90-110^

Ezekiel Bread, Essene Bread
Banana, Mango, Fruit Cocktail, Pineapple
Ice Cream
Green Lentil Soup, Black Bean soup, Pea Soup
Canned Kidney Beans
Orange Juice
Kiwi
Macaroni & Cheese
Oat Bran, Rolled Oats, All Bran
Honey
Corn

70-90^

FOODS	GLYCEMIC INDEX

Vegetables in General not listed above
Fruits in General not listed above
Spaghetti
Pinto Beans
Potato Chips, Chocolate
Oatmeal
Sweet Potatoes, Yams

50-70^

Oranges, Grapes, Yogurt
Navy Beans, Tomato Soup
100% Rye Bread, Cream of Rye Cereal

40-50^

Apples, Pears
Black Eyed Peas, Chick Peas
Milk
Ice Cream
Non-Fat Yogurt

30-40^

Fructose
Lentils
Plums
Peaches
Grapefruit
Cherries

20-30^

Soybeans   **15^**

Peanuts   **12^**

For a more extensive list of specific foods, check Glycemic Index on your computer search engine, or local library.

Note: Meat, Fish, Poultry, and Fat do not affect the Glycemic Index, as they contain no carbohydrates.

TIPS FOR KEEPING THINGS SIMPLE

From my experience in client consultations to lecturing on the subjects of making dietary changes, incorporating a regime of regular exercise or taking dietary supplements, I have learned that most people truly want to feel and look good and enjoy a better quality of life for themselves and their loved ones. I have also learned that most people are somewhat confused as to what vitamins to take, how to shop for healthy foods at the grocery store, or what type of exercise routine is best.

In saying all this, I have come to conclusion that if one can keep their approach to these things as simple as possible, there stands a greater probability for success and so it is with your approach to eating according to your blood type. To further help you understand my point in keeping things simple, try to memorize this statement: "The main thing, is to keep the main thing, the main thing"............ KEEP IT SIMPLE!

In consideration of the varying levels of commitment and tenacity in people, I have listed a few simple and yet realistic tips to follow for long term success. When determining which approach you want to take towards correctly eating foods compatible to your blood type, disregard opinions of others or any outside influences. Simply go by what works best for you. But don't be surprised to find your approach to be blood type influenced.

Choose one of the following approaches:
- SNAIL'S PACE
- ROADRUNNER
- 80% / 20%

SNAIL'S PACE APPROACH

Only a few can jump in head first and make a dramatic 180° dietary turn around and maintain it. But for the rest of the population its a different story. Try not to make all your dietary changes at one time. By simply removing one or two "avoid" foods from your blood type diet and replacing them with food selections from the very beneficial or neutral categories, you will accelerate your results while eliminating unnecessary stress. This approach will contribute to a solid dietary foundation for long term success. Gradually remove another then another "avoid" food from your food choices. By keeping it simple and gradual you will have subtly reached a level of perpetual dietary freedom that will minimize or even eliminate the drop out potential.

ROAD RUNNER'S APPROACH

This approach is short term intended to prove to you what we already know is true in a hurry. For the first 3 weeks do your best to avoid the "avoid" foods for your specific blood type. This will allow your body to begin its detoxification process. As your body detoxifies, you will experience an increase in energy. The body will begin shedding excess body fat. Brain fog will disappear as will bloating and gas from your digestive system. You will begin to enjoy the benefits of stabilized blood sugar levels. You will be well on your way to lowering your blood pressure, cholesterol and preventing the potential of many other health related disorders and diseases. Because you are in a hurry to see results, and are not a true believer yet, you must do this for 3 weeks, then try the following suggestion: For the next 2 days, EAT ONLY AVOID FOODS!

After you do this you will most probably experience:
1. Digestive discomfort, gas, bloating and fatigue.
2. That the answer is truly found in your blood type.

At this point you can decide whether you want to feel that way, one day a week, five days a week or never. The choice is entirely yours!

80% / 20% APPROACH

If you find making dietary changes very challenging, then this approach will help relieve some of the pressure and keep it doable. Simply advance yourself towards making 80% of your food selections from the very beneficial or neutral categories that are listed for your blood type. This in of itself will make you a happier and healthier camper. The remaining 20% of food selections will allow you room for eating foods that you find too difficult to give up. Usually these are those emotional fuzzies or foods that soothe our sweet tooth or cravings. Ironically, as you remain on this approach you will experience less and less of these former cravings that have caused you to get out of control and fail. If you remain faithful at this, you could find yourself moving the percentages up to 85% / 15% because eating correctly for your blood type will eventually become effortless. All of the above approaches are beneficial and effective. Choose which approach best fits you. Play with them and be creative. Learn from the information in the book and how your body responds to the food selections you make. Use this as a measuring tool for making food selections. The premise to this approach to eating foods compatible to your blood type is to make you more aware of how your body will respond to which food you choose to eat. Will your body respond negatively or positively - the choice is yours!

Remember to keep this as simple as you possibly can but most importantly, have fun with it!

Now, to help assist you with losing those unhealthy and unwanted pounds, you will find listed below foods that either contribute to weight loss or cause weight gain per blood type.

BLOOD TYPE "O"

Foods that stimulate weight loss:

Kelp - contains iodine, activates/stimulates thyroid hormone production

Red Meat - revs/stimulates metabolism

Broccoli, Spinach and Kale - stimulates metabolism

Seafood - contains iodine and stimulates thyroid hormone production

Iodized Salt - contains iodine, stimulates thyroid hormone prod.

Liver - stimulates metabolism

Foods that cause weight gain:

Wheat Gluten - slows the metabolism or the metabolic rate ¨

Corn - slows metabolism or slows the metabolic rate ¨

Cauliflower - inhibits thyroid hormone

Brussels Sprouts - inhibits thyroid hormone

Lentils - inhibits improper nutrient metabolism

Navy Beans - poor calorie utilization

Kidney Beans - poor calorie utilization

Cabbage - inhibits thyroid hormone

Mustard Greens - inhibit thyroid production

BLOOD TYPE "A"

Foods that stimulate weight loss:

Vegetable oils - prevent water retention, aids in digestion.

Soy Foods - metabolize quickly and aid in digestion

Vegetables - aid in digestion, increase intestinal mobility

Pineapple - increases calorie utilization, increases intestinal
mobility.

Foods that cause weight gain:

Meat - stores as fat, increases digestive toxins, digests poorly.

Dairy Foods - inhibits nutrient metabolism.

Kidney Beans - slow metabolic rate, interferes with digestive
enzymes.

Lima Beans - slow metabolic rate, interferes with digestive
enzymes.

Wheat (over abundance) - impairs calorie utilization.

BLOOD TYPE "B"

Foods that stimulate weight loss:

Green Vegetables - aids metabolism.

Meat - aids metabolism.

Eggs/Low Fat Dairy - aids metabolism.

Liver - aids metabolism.

Licorice Tea - counters hypoglycemia

Foods that cause weight gain:

Corn - hampers metabolic rate/inhibits insulin efficiency, causes hypoglycemia.

Lentils - cause hypoglycemia, hamper metabolic rate, inhibit proper nutrient uptake.

Peanuts - hamper metabolic efficiency, cause hypoglycemia, inhibit liver function.

Sesame Seeds - hamper metabolic efficiency, cause hypoglycemia.

Buckwheat - inhibits digestion, causes hypoglycemia, hampers metabolic efficiency.

Wheat - slows digestive and metabolic processes, causes foods to store as fat, not to burn as energy, inhibits insulin efficiency.

BLOOD TYPE "AB"

Foods that stimulate weight loss:

Tofu - stimulates metabolic efficiency.

Seafood - promotes metabolic efficiency.

Dairy - improves insulin productivity.

Green Vegetables - improve metabolic efficiency.

Foods that cause weight gain:

Red Meat - stores as fat, poorly digested, toxifies intestinal tract.

Kidney Beans - cause hypoglycemia, slow metabolic rate, inhibit insulin efficiency.

Lima Beans - cause hypoglycemia, slow metabolic rate inhibit insulin efficiency.

Seeds - inhibits insulin efficiency.

Corn - causes hypoglycemia.

Buckwheat - decreases metabolism.

Wheat - decreases metabolism, inefficient use of calories, inhibits insulin efficiency.

NOTE: A drop in blood sugar or hypoglycemia after meals is caused by inhibited insulin production which ultimately leads to less efficient metabolism of foods.

A Final Note

At the beginning of this book the authors stated that many families have members of differing blood types. Probably the most famous family to experience these differences is the Kennedy family, specifically the family of John F. Kennedy, former President of the United States. Without going into great detail, let me illustrate by using a small part of the family tree.

John Francis (Honey Fitz) Fitzgerald -Type O (Wife- Type A)
/
Joseph Kennedy-Blood Type A2 —— Rose Kennedy-Blood Type B
/
Sons:
John F. Kennedy - Blood Type AB
Robert Kennedy - Blood Type A
Ted Kennedy - Blood Type B (unconfirmed)

John F. Kennedy - Type AB —— Jacqueline Kennedy - Type O
/
JFK gave off B gene——JK gave off O gene
/
JFK, Jr. -Blood Type B
Recessive O Gene

John Fitzgerald Kennedy is the only confirmed Blood Type AB president in the history of the United States. He was unique, friendly and adaptable. In fact, during his short presidency, the United States experienced a feeling of national pride and panache that has not been matched to this day. His double dominant genes in conjunction with excellent upbringing and education produced one of our most beloved presidents that this country has ever seen. His influence so great, to this day his grave is visited by millions and his loss to this nation is still mourned. His untimely death is so seared into our psyche, that almost everyone remembers where he or she was, and what he or she was doing at the time of his assassination?

As stated previously, individuals with the AB gene can only pass on the A or B gene, unlike all other blood types that can replicate their genetics. In the present case President John F. Kennedy passed on the B gene. Jacqueline Kennedy, who was Blood Type O, passed on the O gene. In that B is dominant over O, son John F. Kennedy, Jr., was Blood Type B, a different blood type from both his parents. While it is believed that their daughter is also Blood Type B, this has not been confirmed to respect her privacy.

The assertion that JFK, Jr. was different from his father is correct. President Kennedy, true to his blood type, and being very outgoing, loved his life as a politician, unlike his son who was reserved, private, and chose to live out of the limelight. While father welcomed every photo opportunity, the son preferred to pass up the opportunities, and maintain his distance and privacy.

Jacqueline Kennedy, who was Blood Type O and very charismatic and assertive in her own right, would have probably dominated the marriage. However, since JFK was AB, the only blood type to carry two dominant genes, and rarely dominated, she subordinated herself to her husband.

An example of this is Jacqueline's motherly need to shield her children and try to see that they lived a normal life. For this reason, she did not think it appropriate that the press be allowed to photograph the children very often. The President thought differently, but respected her wishes most of the time. However, at times when Jacqueline was away he would invite the presidential photographer for a photo opportunity. He believed that this was good for his personal image, and for his children, consistent with his blood type. It is for this reason that we have many pictures of the children with their father, in the absence of their mother. That famous picture of John, Jr. playing under his father's desk is a prime example. This is not a criticism, but an illustration of how individuals of differing blood type think and act differently.

Years after the assassination Jacqueline went on to marry a man many Americans and others thought unkindly about. Regardless of personal feelings, the one thing Jacqueline had in common with Aristotle Onassis was their blood type, Type O.

Many people reported that JFK, Jr. was a risk taker. This author disagrees. To the contrary, he was a very deliberate, quite, private individual, who gave great thought to his life and actions. He had a great zest for life, and despite suggestions to the contrary, lived life on his own terms out of the public glare.

It is easy to think that someone with his intelligence, money, and celebrity status would want to live a lifestyle in the public eye. But he was his own man who marched to his own drummer, yet not take unnecessary risks. Unconventional, somewhat introverted, but friendly, he chose a private life. His end was the result of inexperience, circumstance, and perhaps bad judgment, a simple human frailty, no more, no less.

JFK, Jr. was a true philanthropist, yet many of his good deeds were achieved without fanfare and publicity. In a short thirty-eight years this noble young prince accomplished much that this country would be proud of for years to come. He was a role model of unselfishness, humility, service to country, and Kennedy values. His untimely death is a tragic loss to his family, his country, and the world.

Many would ask why someone so extremely handsome and likeable, had married so late in life. The answer is in his blood type. Blood Type B is semi-rare and represents about 8% of the world population. Since research has shown blood types are drawn to each other, it was more difficult to find the right mate. In this case, by virtue of his recessive O gene inherited from his mother, JFK, Jr. was obviously drawn to Blood Type O women, his wife included. This does not mean the marriage was wrong, but just accounts for the adjustments the parties are required to make to have a lasting and committed relationship.

Lastly, it was obvious that JFK, Jr. was different from the majority of the Kennedy clan. This is totally consistent considering that with few exceptions, the overwhelming blood types of the remaining Kennedy's are Blood Type A and O respectively.

Regarding the marriage of President Kennedy and Jacqueline Kennedy, it was well known there were difficult times. This is consistent when the two most assertive blood types, AB and O, are themselves. In spite of this fact, no one would deny that both parties were excellent parents. Unfortunately, the difference in blood type of the parties as explained in the Theory of Compatibility espoused in this book, was problematic for both the President and the First Lady.

Many years prior to his marriage to Jacqueline, a young JFK diplomat dated a Swedish woman; also a diplomat named Arvad. The young man and his Swedish friend were deeply in love. But because of circumstances, World War II, and family pressure, young Jack Kennedy was forced to give up this relationship. It took many years to recover from this break-up. Little did he know that this Swedish diplomat was Blood Type AB.

One day President Kennedy met Marilyn Monroe. Yes she was beautiful. Yes, she was a movie star. Yes his actions were unseemly in a legal, ethical, and moral sense, but now that we know she too was rare Blood Type AB, in terms of The Theory of Compatibility, it is explainable.

In a real sense, the lives of individuals take many twists and turns. Until now much has been left to chance in what appears to be random behavior. But now that we know, and research has confirmed, that individuals are drawn to others by blood type traits, it is more understandable. That, which was previously misunderstood, is now clearly visible. There is an answer and reason for everything, and to invoke once again one much wiser than I am:

"God Does Not Play Dice With The Universe"
Albert Einstein

The Answer is in Your Bloodtype

NOTES: